Diagnosis: CANCER
Your Guide Through the First Few Months

Diagnosis: CANCER

YOUR GUIDE THROUGH THE FIRST FEW MONTHS

Wendy Schlessel Harpham, M.D.

Illustrations by Ann Bliss Pilcher

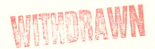

W.W. Norton & Company

New York   London

The text of this book is composed in
11.5/13.5 Berkeley Old Style Book
with the display set in Futura Demi and Futura Bold
Composition and Manufacturing by the Haddon Craftsmen, Inc.
Book design by Margaret M. Wagner

Library of Congress Cataloging-in-Publication Data
Harpham, Wendy Schlessel.
Diagnosis: cancer your guide through the first few months / by Wendy
Schlessel Harpham.
p.   cm.
Includes index.
1. Cancer—Popular works.   2. Cancer—Psychological aspects.
I. Title.
RC263.H36   1992
362.1'96994—dc20   91-37302

ISBN 0-393-03187-X
ISBN 0-393-30892-8 (PBK)

W. W. Norton & Company, Inc.
500 Fifth Avenue, New York, N.Y. 10110
W. W. Norton & Company Ltd.
10 Coptic Street, London WC1A 1PU

1   2   3   4   5   6   7   8   9   0

To Brenda Casey, R.N., John H. Cottey, M.D.,
Susan M. Creagan, M.D., Lizanne Piercy, M.D.,
and James F. Strauss, M.D.

To the families from Congregation Beth Torah and
Presbyterian Hospital of Dallas who helped us

To Ted, Rebecca, Jessica, and William

Contents

Our knowledge about cancer is constantly changing. This book is not intended as a substitute for competent medical care. It serves to supplement the information provided by your doctors and nurses.

Prologue

I was on top of the world at my ten-year medical school reunion. Happily married, the mother of three beautiful children, a successful medical doctor, I enjoyed excellent health. The prior ten years had been devoted to building dreams. I worked hard, often late at night after putting my kids to sleep, but went to the gym three hours per week and was generally home by dinnertime. Weekends "off-call" were usually devoted to my family. My hope was that by balancing my time between hard work, regular exercise, and my family, I would maintain my health and prevent "burn-out."

I left my reunion feeling happy and fulfilled at home and at work, yet daily conscious of the uncertainties of life. Three weeks later I developed excruciating groin and back pain. Two surgeries disclosed disseminated lymphoma, a cancer of the lymph nodes that had spread to many places in my body. The numbing shock, primal fear, and childlike helplessness and dependency stretched each of those first days into what seemed like a week. Facing my own mortality thrust me into a new dimension. Graphic memories of past patients deprived me of the strength and comfort that come from denial. I mentally telescoped my potential futures, focusing on the most frightening of what I had seen the past ten years. As my oncologist gently and dutifully outlined my treatment protocol, my mind reeled with the knowledge of the harm each drug could do, now or later.

Five days after my diagnosis, we started a course of intensive chemotherapy. The next few weeks were a jumble of endless problems, distractions, and responsibilities. My life was turned upside down. Instead of being the person who took care of my family and patients, I was the dependent one, too sick to take care of anyone.

The first step to recovery was accepting that I had become a patient. I had crossed the great divide that separates doctor from patient. Obviously, we are all "patients." But when you deal with illness professionally, day in and day out, you subconsciously create a distance, to the benefit of both the patient being treated and the doctor. Getting cancer shattered this defense mechanism that had allowed me to function effectively as a physician. Once I accepted that I was a patient, I made a conscious effort to be a "good" patient in hopes of maximizing my chances for a smooth and complete recovery. My medical knowledge and experience offered many advantages: the medical settings were all familiar turf, I was secure in the quality of my caretakers, I understood what was happening and why, and I was able to participate in my care. The down side was that I could picture all too vividly the bad things that could happen. Every day that I was sick was a day of strain and worry for my husband, and subtle anxiety for my children. In the short run, I wanted to minimize the pain for my family. In the long run, I wanted to be alive with them and for them as they grew older. My mission became clear: do whatever was required to get well as safely and quickly as possible.

When I was sick, I was two people in one—doctor Harpham and patient Harpham. Doctor Harpham knew what to look for and what a symptom could mean. Patient Harpham, at least in the beginning, was hesitant to report symptoms at a checkup or call my doctors at midnight, because I was self-conscious, a bit embarrassed, and sometimes anxious or afraid. Whenever I hesitated, I recalled my mission to do whatever it took to get well. The disciplined doctor in me governed my actions and overrode the patient's hesitation.

During the months of my chemotherapy, a number of complications developed, some of which required hospitalization. The important point was not that I developed complications, but that all the complications were recognized and reported early. Each hospitalization lasted only two or three days. My doctors were wonderful about responding to my calls and concerns. Problems were nipped in the bud because of my willingness to call my doctors, and their responsiveness and expertise.

While learning how to be a chemotherapy patient, I was overseeing my office. The doctors with whom I shared weekend "call" cared for my patients. For four weeks I used precious time and energy trying unsuccessfully to arrange a substitute physician for my patients. I ended up having to close my practice for ten months. A small group of friends and family came to my home and stuffed two thousand envelopes with "Dear Patient" letters. Mailing that stack of letters was an especially painful loss in the string of losses that began in the emergency room five weeks earlier. Everyone chuckled when my six-year-old daughter responded to a comment about her mommy being a doctor by saying, "Well, my mommy *used* to be a doctor!" I chuckled too, sadly.

Without warning or preparation, I had lost my role as a doctor. Feeling that my world was falling apart, but believing that one can often find good in something that seems bad, I focused on my opportunity to pursue projects and hobbies that had been abandoned. In healthier days, I had frequently day-dreamed about playing my violin. But I consciously had chosen not to play for lack of time. I never doubted that when my children were older, there would be time for my violin. With my medical practice closed, time was *too* abundant, so my violin and I became reacquainted after a ten-year separation. Playing violin was one of my first escapes; improving my vio-lin-playing was one of my first goals; realizing that I could still do things that I enjoyed was one of my first steps towards renewed wholeness. Ironically, being a chemotherapy patient freed me for endeavors not possible as a healthy doctor.

Two months after my diagnosis, my pain was coming under control, the shock was wearing off, and my family was settling into a routine. Playing violin was no longer enough. I started reading everything I could find relating to cancer. I immersed myself in medical texts and journals, pamphlets for patients, trade books on cancer, patient autobiographies, religious books, and books on self-help, positive thinking, meditation, and self-healing. I wanted to know everything there was to know about my cancer, as well as how best to cope with all the unavoidable changes that go with being a cancer patient. I *had* to handle this situation well because my impressionable chil-dren would be learning from me how to be sick, how to interact with the medical profession, and how to cope with a difficult situation. Some of the books were invaluable for their practical information or uplifting message. Other books were awful. They left me feeling that I had caused or contributed signifi-cantly to my cancer, and that I would have to control all future stress if I wanted to get and stay healthy. I had long believed that the emotional and spiritual self affects the physical self, but I could not imagine that they *controlled* all physical happen-ings. My years as a doctor had convinced me that luck, genet-ics, the environment, and a host of greater-than-us factors in-terplayed at the controls of our lives.

One day a friend and I were discussing how much I was

learning from being a patient. She suggested that I write a handout or pamphlet to guide newly diagnosed cancer patients through the initial experience. It was the perfect project. A concise sheet or pamphlet would be excellent for my cancer patients when I returned to work. Over the years I had written short information sheets for my patients to supplement in-office discussions. I have always felt that knowledge helped my patients, because once they understood what was going on they could participate in their own care. Knowledgeable patients helped me because they called with fewer questions and there was a better chance of their following through on my advice. Just as importantly, writing this handout would provide a stimulating "little job" to keep me busy during the weeks that I was isolated because of low white blood cell counts caused by the chemotherapy.

My handout grew and grew as topics were added that I felt would be helpful to patients. At first I just presented facts. Dry, impersonal facts. But having cancer is not impersonal, so I rewrote what I had written and added material, infusing my philosophy about having an illness and dealing with therapy. By the time I finished the original draft, it was book length. This book remained faithful to the original task—it was a relatively concise teaching guide for patients and families. However, a philosophy lay behind it, one grown from experience and reading.

Diagnosis: Cancer Your Guide Through the First Few Months combines my knowledge as a doctor with my experience as a patient. Throughout the book an underlying belief that knowledge brings comfort, hope, and a better chance for improvement or cure is integrated with medical and practical information. The book also grapples with the emotional side of being a cancer patient. As a doctor, I have learned of strength and hope by watching countless brave and graceful patients, people who each day found joy and meaning despite pain or loss. As a patient, I have learned the same lessons through listening to other patients and reading many books. These lessons have been incorporated into the text.

Diagnosis: Cancer Your Guide Through the First Few Months fills an important gap in the literature available to cancer patients. Unlike the numerous books and pamphlets currently available, this is not another cancer patient's story, nor an in-depth medical text, nor a thought-provoking treatise on some aspect of the cancer experience. It is a short and "reader friendly" guide that simplifies the facts, outlines practical issues, and communicates a healthy adaptive philosophy for coping with cancer. This book will help the lay person understand what is happening, participate in his or her care, and adjust to the changes inherent in becoming a cancer patient.

I hope that this book will help other people travel the cancer journey safely and extract the good from their seeming devastation. By leading people away from the gloom of what seems a death sentence and the humiliation of helplessness, I believe that it can direct them towards new meaning and happiness within the constraints of their illness. I also hope that by reviewing all the basics, this book will free doctors and nurses to spend more time answering their patients' specific questions and problems.

Many months have passed since my original diagnosis. My chemotherapy was successful. There is no question that many good things have come out of this unwanted cancer experience. My family and I were the recipients of many people's concern, prayers, time, and energy. I have learned a lot about myself.

I once again wear my white coat. I reluctantly accept that I will wear my patient's gown, too, for the rest of my life. Today I am free of cancer, but I will always be a cancer patient, requiring regular followups to check for recurrent cancer or a complication of my chemotherapy. My experiences as a cancer patient unveiled to me a new appreciation of the fragility of good health, the weaknesses of human nature, and the importance of seizing the moment. This crisis offers me a path to a deeper understanding of my patients and a richer use of my time. I plan on going to my next class reunion. My four-year-old asks me, "are there a lot of days until then?" I answer: "Yes, darling. Many good days."

Introduction

You have just been told that you have cancer. You may be young or old. You may be sick or feel perfectly healthy. You may be recovering from a biopsy or a bigger surgery. Your personal life may be in order or in total disarray. Whatever your situation, your world has just come to a stop. Things are not going to be the way you planned, at least not for the immediate future. Chances are you feel overwhelmed with emotions, information, and responsibilities. It is hard to think clearly. Yet, important decisions need to be made about your medical evaluation and treatment, and your situation at work, school, and home.

This book will help you and your family get through these first few months as easily and safely as possible. It will teach you how to ask the right questions, and make the best decisions *for you* from day one. The philosophy behind this book is that you did not choose to have cancer, but you can choose how you will deal with it. You can choose to cope. Knowledge is good for you. It allows you to participate in your care and be your own best advocate. At the very least, you will understand what is happening to you, even if you want to leave all decision-making to others. Knowledge will help you to regain some control, lessen fear and pain, and look towards your future in a more productive and positive way.

You are not alone. More than one million Americans are diagnosed with cancer each year. *Many millions of people have survived cancer,* and you can learn from them how to get through this transition period. You can learn from their insights and advice without having to discover everything for yourself.

This book offers suggestions for dealing with practical and emotional problems. Only some of the recommendations will apply to you, since this book covers the wide variety of newly diagnosed cancer patients, and everyone is different. This book uses the word "family" to refer to those people who care for you. Your family may be children, parents, siblings, a spouse, a lover, close friends, or other associates. The key is that these people care about you, and are affected by what is happening to you.

You and your family can read this book cover to cover, using whatever information is helpful to you. Or you can skim the chapters for the questions that interest you now. It is common to be so overwhelmed by the diagnosis that you just cannot absorb facts or ideas, so it is a good idea to keep this book handy and reread it periodically the first few months.

You may find it helpful to bring to your doctor a list of your questions, and then write down the answers. It is hard to remember all the questions, let alone to absorb all the answers at the visit with your doctor.

Each section will start off with some bold-print questions, followed by brief answers or outlines of how to get the answer. If you do not know the answer as regards your personal situation, then you should feel free to get the answer from your doctors, nurses, books and pamphlets, or the National Cancer Institute's toll-free information line (1-800-4–CANCER).

Phrases or concepts that can be used as mental tools are printed in boldface as are words defined in the Glossary.

Each topic is addressed more fully in books available at your local bookstore and library. The appendices include a glossary of basic words, a limited annotated bibliography, a brief resource list, a sample medication sheet, an explanation of common tests, an explanation of medical abbreviations, and a sample living will.

Remember:

- Learn as much or as little as you are ready to learn at this time. You do not need to learn or understand everything right away.

- If you do not understand something, there are many places to get the answers, and many people who want to help you to get the answers.

- Every person is unique. Every person's cancer is unique. You need to find out about *your* cancer, and what can be done for you.

- The treatment for cancer is improving daily. Treatments are safer and more effective. There are new ways to minimize side effects, or counteract side effects. Do not let the fear of treatment keep you from getting evaluated or treated.

- We are talking about *your life*. Nothing is more important right now than finding out about your cancer, and making some decisions about how to treat it.

- You can choose how you deal with this new situation.

Acknowledgments

A book like this has many friends who nurtured it from an idea to a working draft to a finished manuscript. Charlotte Loudermilk encouraged the project from its beginning as an idea. A number of people read the first draft with interest and care despite their own hectic schedules: Brenda Casey, R.N., Judi Schlundt, S.W., Becky O'Shea, R.N., Monique Kunkel, M.D., James Strauss, M.D., Billie McAnally, M.D., Stuart Black, M.D., William C. Harvey, M.D., Pam Jenkins, M.S., Edward J. Harpham, Geri Smith, Brenda Kutschke, Judy Koschak, Adele Hess, and Laura Whitehead. Cynthia S. Sherry, M.D. reviewed Appendix E. Linda Houston reviewed the section related to hair loss.

Many people were friends to this book through their support of me and my family. I thank my healthcare team, Brenda Casey, R.N., John H. Cottey, M.D., Susan M. Creagan, M.D., Lizanne Piercy, M.D., and James F. Strauss, M.D., a group of talented people who traversed the treacherous terrain of treating a colleague physician-patient. I thank Rabbi Jeffrey Leynor for teaching and supporting me. I thank Jean and John Harpham for visiting from Delaware a few times, two times on short notice, to care for my children and household. Thanks are also extended to all the caring and generous families from Congregation Beth Torah and Presbyterian Hospital of Dallas who brought meals to our home and helped my husband care for our three children. These efforts enabled me to focus on my treatments, my family, and this book, which was written during the months of my chemotherapy. I thank David A. Cheatham, M.D., and M. Scott Daniel, M.D., who cared for my patients between the time I was diagnosed with lymphoma and the time I temporarily closed my practice. Lastly, I appreciate all the concern and love expressed by family and friends.

Another friend to this book is my editor Mary Cunnane, who came to share in my goal of helping others.

An important friend to this book is my husband, Ted, who not only stayed by my side through all the chemotherapy and hospitalizations, but sacrificed his computer and his study to this project. He reviewed and commented on the manuscript during its various stages of development.

Three young friends to this book are Rebecca, Jessica, and William. They were willing to obey the rules of isolation during the periods of "low white counts" and leave Mommy alone when she was in Daddy's study working on her book.

Diagnosis:
CANCER
Your Guide
Through the
First Few
Months

—

1

Understanding Cancer

DIAGNOSIS AND STAGING

What Is Cancer?

Cancer is a very general term that refers to more than two hundred different diseases (types of cancer). All types of cancer

- have uncontrolled growth of cells;
- can spread through the blood and lymph (a clear fluid that circulates in the body) to other parts of the body.

Each type of cancer is different, and you need to find out about your type of cancer in order to understand your situation. There are different treatments for each type of cancer. Some cancers are very slow-growing, and do not cause problems for a long time. Some cancers are very fast-growing (aggressive) and cause serious problems if not treated immediately. Some cancers are usually curable, some are rarely curable. Some cancers usually spread to other parts of the body (e.g., bone, brain, lung), some cancers rarely spread or only spread late.

Am I Going to Die?

Cancer is not a death sentence, it is an illness. Nearly half of all people diagnosed with cancer will be *cured* with treatment. Almost half of all people diagnosed with cancer will be alive five years after their diagnosis. Many cancers are not curable, but are still treatable, allowing the person to live a relatively normal life much like someone with a chronic illness such as diabetes. Rarely, a person's cancer will disappear without any treatment (a "spontaneous **remission**").

The usual course of events is that without treatment cancer continues to grow, eventually blocking the body's normal functions and causing death.

Am I Going to Have Pain?

Most people with cancer have no pain when the cancer is early. Even in late stages, less than half of the patients have significant pain due to the cancer.

Pain can be controlled. There are many safe, effective ways to control pain. If you keep your doctor informed about any pain, you can work together to get your pain under control (see section on pain control, p. 58).

What Is My Prognosis?

Prognosis is the prediction of how you will do (how long you will live, what problems you will have). Your prognosis depends on

- your type of cancer;
- how far advanced your cancer is;
- your physical fitness;
- the presence or absence of any other medical conditions;
- many factors that we cannot measure (e.g., your "will to live").

A prognosis is an educated guess based on statistics, and nobody can predict exactly how *you* will do. Your doctor can give you some idea of how serious your immediate and long-term situation is. Knowing this will help you and your family prepare for whatever is ahead of you.

New and improved treatments become available regularly. The statistics that help determine your prognosis are based on the best information that doctors have. However, it is impossible to give long-range information on therapy that has only been used with patients for a short time. In many cases, your prognosis is actually much better than what the numbers suggest.

Your prognosis does not determine how you as an individual will do. There are individuals who have been cured of every type of cancer. Every type of cancer can be treated in some way.

Is Cancer Contagious?

No, cancer is not contagious. You did not catch it from anyone, and you cannot give it to anyone by close contact.

If you spend time with children, it is very important to make it clear to them right away that your condition is not contagious. If this is not said outright, these children could worry that they will catch it from you if they are close to you, or that they caused you to get sick. One way to explain cancer is likening it to a broken bone, a cut, or a headache. "Just like you cannot catch a broken leg, you cannot catch cancer."

How Did I Get This Cancer?

Our bodies are made up of billions of cells which divide in order to grow and repair the body. We are constantly making new hair, blood, skin, bone, and so on. It is believed that cancer starts as a loss of control of one, single cell. Over time—sometimes months, but often years—the cancer grows big enough to be detectable or cause problems.

We are learning more and more about how that first cell gets out of control and how cancers get started. We know that some things increase the risk (the chance) of getting certain cancers. However, many people with these risk factors do not ever get cancer, and many people with no known risk factors do get cancer. It is very probable that more than one thing has to go wrong to cause cancer to start.

Cancer is not caused by injuring yourself (e.g., bumping your breast, or leg, or testicle). An injury may bring a cancer to your attention, but the injury did not cause the cancer.

It is natural to look for a cause for your cancer, and to search your past for an explanation of "what you did wrong." From a practical point of view, **Now is not the time to spend looking for a cause for your cancer:**

- Finding the cause will not make your cancer go away
- You cannot change anything that you did in the past
- Blaming yourself does not help anyone or anything
- Time and energy spent looking for a cause is time taken away from dealing with today and deciding what to do next

Am I Putting My Family at Risk for Cancer If I Do Not Look for a Cause of My Cancer?

Some cancers have a tendency to run in families. Discuss with your doctor if your family members need to be evaluated in any special way. Some cancers are related to known environmental exposures. Again, discuss with your doctor if your family needs to pursue evaluation of their environment, or undergo any special screening tests.

These are issues that can usually wait until the flurry surrounding your evaluation has settled down. Do not let a search for a cause delay your evaluation and treatment.

Did Stress Cause My Cancer?

Stress does not cause cancer. Most doctors and patients believe that stress does play an important role in your health. When people are diagnosed with cancer after a particularly stressful time, they may be inclined to blame the stress. Although the stress may have played a role in when the cancer became more active, the stress did not cause the cancer. Many people lead very, very stressful lives and never develop cancer.

You cannot change anything that you did in the past. After you get through this initial adjustment phase, you can and should pay attention to how much stress you have in your life, and how you want to deal with your stress from now on. Dealing with stress in a healthy way may improve your chances for a good response to your therapy. Even if it does not improve your chances, your life will be happier and more comfortable.

Did My Diet Cause My Cancer?

Many foods have been reported to cause cancer. It is difficult to prove causation. Some foods and dietary habits have been shown to be associated with an increased risk of cancer. Among them are:

- Heavy alcohol consumption, associated with cancers of the liver, throat, esophagus, and mouth. The risk is increased greatly if the person also smokes.
- High dietary fat is associated with cancers of the colon, rectum, breast, uterus, prostate, testes, gallbladder.
- Nitrites (smoked or salted fish, dried fish, pickled vegetables) are associated with cancers of the stomach and esophagus.
- Aflatoxins (spoiled peanuts) are associated with liver cancer.
- Low levels of vitamins A and C are associated with cancers of the esophagus, stomach, colon, rectum, prostate, bladder, lung, larynx.

Even if your diet was the type of diet associated with an increased risk for your type of cancer, it is still very difficult to determine how much your diet contributed to your cancer. All of the information on diet is related to groups of people, not individuals.

Is My Cancer Related to AIDS?

People with AIDS (acquired immune deficiency syndrome) are at increased risk of

- **Kaposi's sarcoma**
- intermediate and high-grade **non-Hodgkin's lymphoma**

An AIDS blood test may be discussed if you have Kaposi's sarcoma or a high-grade lymphoma.

Does Having Cancer Put Me at Increased Risk for Getting AIDS?

No. As far as is known, you have the same risk of getting AIDS as you did prior to your diagnosis of cancer. If your cancer therapy requires you to receive blood products, there is a very small risk of transfusion-associated infection.

What Is My Diagnosis? What Type of Cancer Do I Have?

Your **diagnosis** is the name of your illness, in this case the name of your cancer. The only way to make a definite diagnosis of cancer is by getting a piece of tissue, and examining it under the microscope. A specialized doctor, called a **pathologist**, can usually determine what kind of cancer you have by how the cells look under the microscope. Thyroid cancer cells look like altered thyroid cells, lung cancer cells look like altered lung cells.

The name of a cancer is based on where the cancer first started, if this can be determined. A cancer in the lung that started in the lung is a "lung cancer." A cancer in the lung that started in the breast is a "breast cancer" that spread to the lung.

Cancer that started in the lung looks like lung cancer under the microscope, no matter where the sample of tissue was taken from. If you have lung cancer that spread to the bone, the cancer cells in your lung look the same as the cancer cells in your bone. Each cancer is classified under one of the following groups:

- **carcinoma**: cancer that started in the lining and covering tissues of organs or ducts
- **sarcoma**: cancer that started in the soft tissue (muscles, nerves, tendons, blood vessels) or bone
- **lymphoma**: cancer of the lymph system
- **leukemia**: cancer of the white blood cells
- **multiple myeloma**: cancer of the plasma cells in the bone marrow

Why Is My Diagnosis So Important?

Since each type of cancer is really a separate disease, your diagnosis needs to be as accurate as possible, so that you are getting treated for the right disease. Your diagnosis is a key factor in determining what your **prognosis** is, and what treatment options are available.

Is My Cancer Malignant?

- **malignant** = cancer
- **benign** = not cancer, not malignant
- **tumor** = abnormal growth = neoplasm = benign or malignant
- **lesion** = abnormal area = benign or malignant

When doctors use the term "cancer", they are referring to a malignant tumor. A "tumor" is any overgrowth of cells, benign or malignant. "Malignant" means that the tumor can spread (metastasize). If a malignant cancer is not controlled, it eventually interferes with the body's normal functions (breathing, digestion, waste elimination) and leads to death.

A benign tumor cannot spread. It can cause problems if it grows near a vital structure, but it is rarely life-threatening. Technically speaking, there is no such thing as a "benign cancer."

Is There Any Uncertainty about My Diagnosis?

Usually the diagnosis is definite, and no matter how many different doctors read your biopsy slides, they will all agree as to the type of cancer. Sometimes the diagnosis is not certain. This can happen even if everything is done perfectly, because of the nature of your particular cancer cells. When the diagnosis is at all uncertain, your slides should be read by several doctors, hopefully some of whom have special expertise in your type of cancer.

What Is the "Primary Lesion"?

The place where a cancer starts, where the first cell got out of control, is called the primary site. The cancer that is in the primary site is called the **primary lesion**. Cancers are named after the primary site, even if they have spread to other places (e.g., as I mentioned, cancer that started in the colon and spread to the liver is still "colon" cancer). Sometimes the cancer in the primary site is very small, or even undetectable, but we know that the cancer started there because of what the cancer cells look like under the microscope.

How Big Is My Primary Lesion?

The size of the primary lesion is sometimes a factor that helps determine the prognosis, the urgency in treatment, and the options for therapy.

What Does It Mean to "Metastasize"? What Is a Metastasis?

To **metastasize** is to travel or spread. When cells from the primary (original) cancer break off and spread to another part of the body through the blood or the lymph, they are said to have metastasized. All cancers can metastasize. The cancer at the new site is called a **metastasis**.

Under the microscope, all of your cancer cells look like each other, no matter where they are (i.e., if you have cancer in the lung, and liver, and bone, the cells from each area look alike under the microscope).

What If My Doctors Tell Me That They Do Not Know Where the Cancer Started?

Sometimes all the doctors agree with the type of your cancer (e.g., **carcinoma**), but they cannot tell where your cancer started (e.g., breast, colon, lung). This is because even with our current technology, it is impossible to know. This is called a "cancer of unknown primary" or "cancer of unknown origin." There are routine procedures for evaluating and treating this situation.

After I Have a Diagnosis, What Is the Next Step?

After you have been diagnosed with cancer through a biopsy or surgery, your doctors perform additional tests to

- determine what stage your cancer is in (see next three questions);
- evaluate for any changes or problems caused by your cancer;
- evaluate your general medical condition unrelated to the cancer.

What Is Staging?

Staging is the evaluation to find out

- how big your cancer is;
- if and where your cancer has spread;
- if there are any problems being caused by your cancer.

A stage is meaningful only when interpreted for a specific type of cancer. "Stage 3" for one cancer does not have the same implications as "stage 3" for another cancer. Each type of cancer has its own criteria for determining which stage the cancer is in. There are a number of different staging systems. The higher the stage, the more advanced the cancer.

How Is Staging Done?

Obtaining information about your cancer through tests is called "**staging**." Staging is done by

- talking to you (taking a history);
- doing a physical exam;
- doing various tests and studies;
- sometimes performing surgery.

When you are undergoing tests, you are "being staged." The results of all the tests tells the doctor what "stage" your cancer is in.

Why Is Staging Important?

Cancers of the same type and in the same stage tend to follow the same course. Therefore, knowing the stage of your cancer helps

- determine your prognosis;
- plan your therapy;
- evaluate your response to therapy.

Keep in mind that many factors other than cancer type and stage determine how you will do. As advances are made in our understanding of **oncology**, other factors such as **hormone status, receptor expression**, and **biochemical markers** are becoming important.

What Are the Options Regarding My Staging?

Sometimes there are options regarding how and how much to evaluate. One doctor may suggest surgery to evaluate for lymph nodes in the abdomen, whereas another doctor may recommend non-invasive scans (pictures) to get the same in-

formation. This is where another opinion is particularly helpful. If all options seem reasonable, then other factors will determine the decision (convenience of location, trust in doctor).

In What Stage Is My Cancer?

Your doctor can tell you what stage your cancer is in after
performing some tests (see prior four questions).

Do I Really Need to Have All These Tests?

Your doctors need to know as much as they can about your
individual cancer and your overall medical condition because:

• General predictions about your cancer can be made based
on the stage of your cancer;

• Most treatment options are based on the stage of your cancer
and your medical condition;

• Potential problems or complications may be picked up that
can be minimized or avoided;

• Doctors follow the response of your cancer to any treatments by rechecking these tests after treatment. For example, if you have a spot on your X ray or scan now, and the
spot disappears after treatment, then your doctors can usually conclude that the cancer disappeared at that spot.

Has My Cancer Spread (Metastasized)?

Tests are done to determine if your cancer has spread (**metastasized**). If a test shows an abnormal spot, then it is possible
that the cancer has spread to that area. The only way to prove

that any abnormality is cancer is to get a piece of it (i.e., biopsy it) and look at it under the microscope. Your doctors can tell you how sure they are that any spots are cancer, or are not cancer.

What Is a "Negative" Test Result?

- negative = normal = not abnormal = not cancer
- positive = not normal = abnormal = possibly cancer or definitely cancer (depending on the test)

A test result is called "negative" when the results are normal.

In general terms, when a test result is negative, the test shows no potentially active abnormalities (e.g., a chest X ray with no evidence of fluid in the lung, or heart disease, or a spot in the lung, or fractured ribs).

When discussing a test result with reference to your cancer diagnosis, negative means no evidence of cancer. For example, a chest X ray with no evidence of cancer could show abnormalities, such as an enlarged heart, but it is still negative for cancer.

What Is a Positive Test Result?

A test result is called "positive" when the results are not normal.

In general terms, when a test result is positive, the test shows some active abnormality, such as the chest X ray with evidence of fluid in the lung, and so on. The abnormality could be due to cancer or to a problem totally unrelated to cancer.

When discussing a test result with reference to your cancer

diagnosis, "positive" means an abnormality that may be cancer or is cancer. A chest X ray is called positive if it has a new spot in the lung. Further tests may prove whether this spot is benign (not cancer) or malignant (cancer).

When discussing the results of a biopsy with reference to your cancer, "positive" means cancer.

If My Test Is "Negative" or "Good," Does This Guarantee That My Cancer Has Not Spread to the Area Tested?

No. A negative or normal test result is reassuring, but does not guarantee that you are cancer-free in the area being tested. If a cancer is too small, it cannot be detected by these tests. For example, a **CAT scan** (also called a CT scan, a sophisticated X ray) of the liver can pick up spots that are one-half centimeter (approximately one-quarter inch) or bigger in diameter. A normal CAT scan tells you that it is unlikely that there are any areas of cancer one-half centimeter or bigger. Nevertheless, there may be spots of cancer smaller than one-half centimeter in that area.

How Quickly Is My Cancer Growing?

Doctors estimate how quickly your cancer is growing based on

- what the cells look like under the microscope;
- the history of similar cancers (i.e., statistics);
- your history (e.g., the lump has doubled in size in one month versus six months).

By looking at your cells under the microscope, doctors can see how closely your cancer cells look like mature, normal cells. If the cancer cells look mature, then they are called "well-differentiated." In general, these tend to be slower-growing cancers. If the cancer cells look very immature, then they are called "undifferentiated" or "poorly differentiated." In general, these are faster-growing cancers. Another phrase you may hear is "high-grade" (fast-growing) or "low grade" (slow-growing).

- well-differentiated = low-grade = slow-growing
- poorly differentiated = high-grade = fast-growing

How Quickly Does My Staging Need to Be Done?

Your medical condition may necessitate a speedy evaluation and early treatment. More often than not, you have some time to gather your support group, and find out about your cancer.

Always keep in mind that every day that you are not being treated, your cancer is continuing to grow. For many cancers, the earlier you start treatment, the better your chance for success.

Timely, thorough staging is important because

- treatment is based on staging; you usually cannot start treatment until you complete the staging;
- some staging procedures (e.g., surgery) will cause a delay in treatment, so the longer you delay the staging, the longer you are delaying the treatment of your cancer;
- if you begin treatment before the staging is complete, then you may lose a marker—a test indicating presence of cancer—that could have been followed after treatment. For example, if you have an X ray during or after treatment that shows a spot, you will not know if the spot is new (i.e., you are not responding to therapy), or smaller (i.e., you are responding), or unchanged (i.e., you are being controlled, but you may need a change in therapy).

TREATMENT

Why Do We Treat Cancer?

There are four reasons to treat cancer:

- To relieve pain or other symptoms
- To prevent complications from the cancer
- To prevent or slow progression of the cancer
- To cure the cancer

What Is a Remission?

A **remission** is when there is no detectable sign of your cancer. You may have no detectable sign of your cancer after surgery (even before planned chemotherapy or radiation therapy), or during the course of your treatments, or at the end of treatment. Many patients achieve a complete remission, only to have the same cancer show up again months or years later. You must achieve a complete remission and maintain the remission for a specified amount of time before you are considered **cured.**

What Is a "Response" or a "Partial Remission"?

You have shown a "response" or a "partial remission" when your cancer responds to treatment by shrinking at least in half but there are still signs of cancer. Some people may use the terms "response" or "partial remission" when there is *any* shrinkage of your cancer. Clarify with your doctors what they mean if they use these terms.

What Is a Recurrence?

You are said to have a **recurrence** if you have been treated for cancer in the past with complete disappearance of all evidence of cancer, and now there is evidence that the same cancer has come back.

What Is a ''Cure''?

When doctors talk of a cancer **cure**, they usually mean that there is no detectable sign of cancer and the person has the same life expectancy as if he or she never had cancer. Sometimes doctors use the word "cure" when there is no evidence of cancer for at least five years. This is because for most cancers five years is a fairly reliable time after which the chance of recurrence is extremely low. Some cancers can be called cured in one year, other cancers cannot be called cured even after five years with no sign of cancer. Every cancer is different. You will need to find out what your doctors mean when they talk about curing your type of cancer.

What Are the Treatment Options for My Cancer?

Conventional and most investigational treatments involve

- medicines (**chemotherapy, hormonal therapy**);
- surgery;
- radiation;
- **immunotherapy (biological therapy)**;
- some combination of the above.

The specific options for your treatment depend on

• your diagnosis;

• the stage of your cancer;

• your general medical health, other than your cancer.

What Is Chemotherapy (Chemo)?

Chemotherapy is the use of chemicals to treat a disease. Technically speaking, all chemical medicines (e.g., antibiotics, blood pressure medicines, pain medicines) are chemotherapy. However, when we say "chemotherapy," we are usually talking about medicines to kill cancer cells. **Hormone therapy** is included in this group.

Chemotherapy can be given by mouth (pills) or by injection into a vein (intravenous), artery, or muscle. Occasionally, the medicines are injected directly into spinal fluid, into an artery supplying a cancer, or into another part of the body.

The word "chemotherapy" is very scary to many people. Think of chemotherapy as medicine to treat your cancer the same way antibiotics treat infection. Some chemotherapy is very mild and well-tolerated. Other chemotherapy regimens are rough. The big advantage of chemotherapy is that it is systemic, i.e., it treats the entire system or body. When there is reason to believe that you may have cancer cells that cannot be reached with surgery or radiation, chemotherapy has the best chance of killing cancer cells anywhere in your body.

What Is Radiation Therapy?

Radiation therapy is also called radiotherapy, or irradiation therapy. It includes:

- External radiation: using a machine that aims a high-energy beam at spot(s) known to be cancer
- Internal radiation: giving a radioactive source by injection or mouth
- Interstitial radiation (brachytherapy): inserting "seeds" of radiation in or near a cancer, either temporarily or permanently

The radiation kills the cancer cells. Radiation is used to cure some cancers, and control pain in other cancers. It is also used to shrink cancers before surgery, or "clean up" any leftover cancer cells in an area after surgery.

Therapy has improved over the past years, so that lower doses of radiation are used. Radiation therapy is now more accurate. There is less damage to normal tissue, and therefore there are fewer side effects than there used to be. The advantages of radiation are:

- Radiation can reach areas that cannot be reached with surgery;
- Radiation usually requires a shorter course of therapy than chemotherapy;
- Radiation may be an option in people who have medical conditions that rule out surgery or chemotherapy as treatment possibilities;
- There are fewer physical changes than with some surgery (e.g., removal of all or part of a breast) or chemotherapy (e.g., hair loss).

The disadvantages of radiation are:

- Radiation usually requires a greater time investment than surgery;

RADIATION TREATMENT

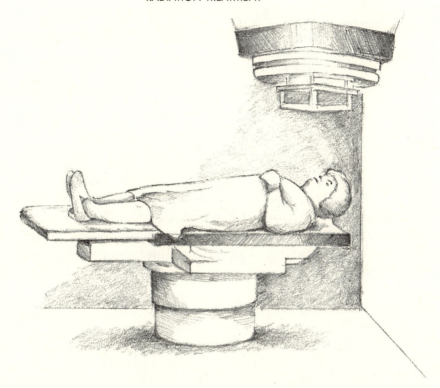

The patient is left alone in the shielded room during the few minutes it takes to deliver the dose of radiation. Technicians and doctors communicate with the patient via two-way intercom.

- Radiation can only kill cancer cells in the field of treatment;
- Radiation is available only at hospitals and at cancer treatment centers.

What Is Biological Therapy (Immunotherapy)?

Immunotherapy is a new, experimental approach to treating cancer. It involves giving medicines that will boost your own immune system to fight the cancer. It includes

- interferon
- interleukin
- CSFs (colony stimulating factors)
- TNFs (tumor necrosis factors)
- monoclonal antibodies

Are My Treatment Options Standard?

A treatment option is standard when it is recommended routinely. Standard therapy comes out of years of well-controlled studies and is felt to be relatively safe and effective. Doctors can provide information on the risks, side effects, and chances of success for each standard therapy. Advantages of standard therapy include:

- Doctors have more experience with it, so they can prepare you for what is involved;
- It is available at most facilities that treat cancer patients;
- It is usually covered by insurance.

What Is Investigational Treatment?

When a drug or a treatment is under study, it is called "investigational" or "experimental." Oncologists around the world are conducting studies on patients using

- new combinations of old drugs or treatments;
- completely new drugs or treatments;
- new drugs or treatments in combination with old drugs or treatments.

What Are Clinical Trials?

After investigation has shown a drug or treatment to have some anti-tumor effect in lab tests, it is studied in trials involving human patients. These investigational studies, called "clinical trials," are aimed at finding safer and more effective treatments for all the different types of cancer. With time, the successful treatments in the clinical trials become the new standard treatment.

In the United States, clinical trials are overseen by

- the National Cancer Institute, or
- a "cooperative group," an organized group of oncologists from a number of hospitals and clinics, who are trained in designing, running, and interpreting clinical trials, or
- a qualified individual oncologist or group of oncologists in one institution or clinic.

There are three different kinds of clinical trials. The earliest trials, "phase 1" trials, are designed to determine the safety of a new treatment. These trials are reserved for a few people with very advanced cancers who have little hope of relief or cure with standard therapy. When a medication or treatment has been shown to be safe, it can be given in phase 2 trials. These trials involve larger numbers of people and are designed to determine if these treatments are effective against specific types of cancer. When a treatment has been shown to be safe and effective, it enters phase 3. Phase 3 trials are designed to determine if a new treatment is better than standard therapy.

How Can I Find Out Which Clinical Trials Are Available?

It is best to find out about clinical trials from your doctors. Your doctors can find out about available clinical trials related to your cancer by contacting:

- PDQ (Physician Data Query), a frequently updated computerized list of trials in progress related to all kinds of cancer, a service of the National Cancer Institute, the network of oncologists involved in clinical trials around the country. These oncologists are aware of ongoing trials that are not registered with the NCI's PDQ.

Should I Consider Investigational Treatment?

You should consider investigational treatment if:

- You have a rare cancer
- Your chances for cure or good response are very low with standard therapy
- You live near a cancer center that is conducting clinical trials

The main advantage to investigational therapy is that it may prove to be the best treatment for you, giving you the best chance for a good outcome. The disadvantages include:

- Less predictability of success (however, success is usually at least as likely as with standard treatment except in very early studies)
- Restricted availability (only available at certain centers)

- Possible problems with insurance reimbursement (although some clinical trials will treat you at no charge)
- Physician referral needed

Can I Be Treated with Investigational Therapy Without My Knowing It?

No. All investigational therapy requires written "informed consent" before beginning any treatments.

Do I Have Any Other Options If Standard Therapy Offers Me Very Little Hope of Improvement or Cure, AND I Am Not a Candidate for Any Clinical Trials, OR There Are NO Ongoing Clinical Trials for My Cancer Situation?

If you have a very serious cancer, and the chance for improvement or cure is very low with currently available treatment:

- You may be a candidate for a drug or treatment that your doctor can get for you under the FDA's "compassionate use" guidelines. These drugs are very new; their safety and efficacy are less certain, but they may offer you more hope than standard therapy.
- You can call the major cancer centers and inquire if they are conducting any trials for your cancer that are not registered with NCI.

When *all* treatment options in the United States leave one in a hopeless situation, some people contact one of the private enterprises who, for a fee, will provide a list of trials and treatments available worldwide, outside of the American medical mainstream. **This should be an option of last resort when in an otherwise hopeless situation.** Most oncologists discourage this option.

Before making any treatment decisions, discuss your findings about treatment options with your doctor.

Why Are Some Treatments Only Available Outside of the United States?

In addition to standard American medical treatments, and treatments involved in clinical trials, treatments are being given outside the American medical mainstream. These treatments are not subject to the same stringent regulation as in the United States. The main reasons for the regulation in the United States are:

- To protect you from ineffective treatment, especially when effective treatment is available
- To protect you from dangerous treatment, especially when less dangerous treatment is available
- To protect you from unscrupulous individuals who want to exploit you for financial gain

An unintended consequence of strict American regulation is that a superior new treatment might become available outside of the United States before it is available here.

There are many practical problems inherent in being treated outside of the American medical mainstream, such as:

- Difficulty finding an American doctor to administer the treatments

- Need to travel, often far distances (expense, separation from support group, possible language problem)
- Possible problems with insurance reimbursement

What Is Alternative Treatment?

Alternative or unconventional therapy is treatment that has been shown by the medical profession to be ineffective at best, and possibly harmful. Examples include laetrile (the apricot pit medicine), herbal tonics, and "metabolic therapy." These treatments have been well-investigated. If these alternative treatments were as good as conventional therapy, as documented by scientific research, they would be used in conventional therapy. Some people are attracted to alternative therapy because:

- They find the risks and side effects of conventional therapy too frightening
- They are discouraged if they have a cancer that is difficult to treat with conventional therapy
- They have had unpleasant experiences with conventional medical doctors in the past
- They find the doctors involved with alternative therapy more encouraging and/or more supportive than the conventional medical doctors whom they have seen for their cancer

The most important decision that you will make in the immediate future is what type of treatment you will take. If you proceed with treatment that is ineffective or harmful, you will lose valuable time that could make a major difference in your future. Some doctors will assist you in pursuing alternative therapy in addition to conventional therapy. The doctors should make sure that the alternative therapy does not counteract or interfere with the conventional therapy.

What Is Supplemental Therapy?

Supplemental treatment options include visual imagery, special diets, prayer, and relaxation. These can become an important part of your therapy. These therapies should not be used as your only therapy. Books, nurses, and support groups can teach you about these therapies.

Where Can Treatment Be Given?

Any location is only as good as the treatment available and the doctors working there. You must consider the doctor's expertise in the type of cancer that you have.

Your treatment may last a long time (many months to years) so the closer to home that you can receive treatments, the easier it will be. Some people start their treatments in a large medical center, and continue their treatments in a more local medical facility. Some treatments will only be available at certain hospitals or centers.

What Is the Difference between In-patient and Out-patient Treatment?

The terms "in-patient" and "out-patient" are administrative terms.

"In-patient" refers to any treatment given to you after you have been officially admitted to a hospital. Your care is expected to require at least an overnight stay.

"Out-patient" refers to any care given in an office, clinic, or hospital that is administered to you when you are signed in as an out-patient.

Insurance policies frequently reimburse differently depending on whether a treatment is administered on an in-patient or out-patient basis. Find out about your insurance coverage, and discuss this with your doctor when planning treatment.

What Are the Risks of Each Treatment Option?

The risks are:

- Side effects: unfavorable symptoms or changes from therapy that are expected (such as nausea, hair loss, sore mouth, fatigue)
- Complications: problems that arise from therapy (such as infection, dehydration, phlebitis) and that threaten your health or life

Some complications, if they occur, happen during treatment (e.g., infection). Other complications, if they occur, appear long after treatment is completed (e.g., second cancers, leukemia, blocked bowels from scarring). Some complications are quite predictable, and you can be monitored closely so as to minimize the risk (e.g., anemia). Some complications are very unpredictable, and can only be treated after they occur. Some complications are easy to treat and are rarely a threat to your health or life (e.g., rash). Other complications are very serious (infection, bleeding).

The risk of each treatment option will depend on

- which treatment is used;
- your type of cancer;
- how advanced your cancer is;
- the presence or absence of any other medical conditions (e.g., heart, lung, or kidney problems).

Remember that everyone is different. Statistics cannot predict which problems, if any, you will have with any given course of treatment. **Millions of people have tolerated these treatments, and now enjoy healthy lives.**

Talking about the risks of cancer treatment can be frightening. That is because the risks are being laid out in front of you, and you are concentrating on them. You deal with risk all the time, but you usually do not focus on it. For example, when you apply for your first driver's license, chances are that you are excited about your new ability to come and go more freely. You know that you will have the inconvenience of driver's education classes and the driver's test. There will be new expenses (license, insurance). You also know that there are real risks to your health and life every time you drive. But the advantages are so great that the inconveniences, expense, and long-term risks are worth it. Once you make your decision to get a license, you do not think about all the risks, and you put all of your energy into driving.

Treatments offer you a way to improvement or cure. Treatments and their risks must be seen as good. Some treatments are risky because they are strong therapies that work. After you weigh the risks of a treatment and make your decision, focus on the benefits of the chosen treatment.

What Are the Advantages of Each Treatment Option?

Treatments can have advantages in terms of:

- Better cure rates, or better response rates
- Fewer side effects
- Less short-term risk
- Less long-term risk

- Less expense
- More experience with the treatment (doctors have more experience with a treatment that has been used for many years than a treatment that is new)
- Local availability

Will My Age Affect My Treatment Options?

Age does affect treatment options. Treatment is given to improve overall quality of life and to prolong life, but it can also hurt the quality of life and risk shortening life.

- One issue is whether, at your age, aggressive treatment would really add more quality or quantity of life than less aggressive treatment. (For a ninety-year-old person with a slow-growing cancer, he or she may have the same life expectancy with a much better quality of life with less aggressive treatment than with aggressive treatment.)
- Normal, unavoidable, age-associated changes in your body make some treatments too risky after a certain age. For example, most transplant centers feel that bone marrow transplant is too risky for someone over sixty years old, no matter how excellent his or her physical condition.

How True Are All the Unpleasant Stories about Therapy?

Advances in cancer therapy include strides in preventing or decreasing the side effects of therapy. There are support groups and self-help books that can teach you how to minimize side effects and deal well with them if you have them.

If you hear unpleasant stories, remember:

- If a person was treated more than a year ago, he or she did not have the same medicines to deal with side effects as are currently available. An excellent anti-nausea medicine became available in the spring of 1990.

- If a person received different treatment or has a different cancer, you can expect a different experience.

Even if everything about the other person is similar (same age and sex patient, same type of cancer, same stage of cancer, same therapy, same general health), you are still a different person. The response to therapy is very individual. Like many other experiences, your attitude makes a difference. For example, if you go into chemotherapy expecting to be very sick, you probably will be. If you go into it with a positive attitude, you have a better chance of milder symptoms.

If I Do Not Have Many Side Effects, Is My Therapy Working?

Yes. Many people have few or no significant side effects from their therapy, and have an excellent response of their cancer. The effect of therapy on your cancer is not reflected in your side effects.

How Quickly Does My Treatment Need to Be Started?

If you are having symptoms from your cancer, or you have a very fast-growing cancer, then you will probably need to get started on treatment quickly. If you were diagnosed by a biopsy of a painless lump, then you probably have some time to make your decision. Your doctors will be able to advise you how much time you have to decide on therapy.

Therapy is a big commitment in terms of time, energy, emotions, and money. It is wise to invest the time and energy into researching with your doctor what is the best treatment plan *for you*. On the other hand, your cancer will continue to grow until treatment is started. *If you spend too much time delaying or researching, you may be losing valuable treatment time.*

Will My Evaluation or Treatment Affect My Ability to Have Children, Now or Later?

Although future fertility may be the farthest thing from your mind right now, you need to address it so that in the future you do not regret any decisions you make now. You want to be able to look back and know that you made informed decisions.

Some tests and treatments affect the ability of a man to produce sperm, or the ability of a woman to get pregnant or have a normal pregnancy. Some tests and treatments raise concerns about the risks to the unborn child conceived or carried during tests and treatment.

If there is any chance that you are pregnant, tell your doctors immediately.

Are There Any Precautions I Can Take to Minimize the Risk to My Fertility?

There are ways to minimize the risk to your fertility:

- When there are equally good alternative tests and treatments, choose the option that carries the least risk regarding fertility.
- Inquire whether any of your tests and treatments can be done with extra shielding.

• If you are a woman about to undergo surgery or radiation to your abdomen, inquire whether you are a candidate for tacking your ovaries out of the field of intended radiation, thus decreasing exposure of your eggs to radiation.

Can I Save ("Bank") My Sperm or Eggs?

If there is concern that future fertility may be impaired, you should discuss saving your sperm or (fertilized) eggs before you receive any treatments. You may want to contact a medical center or physician specializing in fertility to get the most up-to-date information.

What Is Access?

Access refers to any connection into your bloodstream. Access is needed:

• To get blood samples from you
• To give medicines to you
• To give fluids to you
• To give blood to you

Types of access (explained below) include:

• Peripheral access (I.V.)
• Central access (Groshong or Hickman catheter, central line, ports)
• Pumps

What Is an I.V.?

"I.V." stands for "intravenous," or "in the vein." "Peripheral access" is a fancy term for the usual I.V. catheter in your hand or arm. This allows fluids or medications to be given directly into your blood. It should be changed every three days or so. Two advantages of I.V. therapy over oral (by mouth) therapy are:

• Some medications are only available as I.V. medications;

• I.V. medications and fluids can be given when someone is unable to eat, or when digestion is not working normally.

What Is a Groshong Catheter? What Is a Hickman Catheter?

These are tubes (catheters) that enter the body near the heart. They are placed by a surgeon under local or general anesthesia. The advantages are:

• You can receive blood, fluids, and medicines repeatedly without discomfort

• You can give blood samples repeatedly without discomfort

• The catheter can be left in place for weeks to months

• The catheter is easy to use and easy to remove

The disadvantages are:

• The risks associated with placing the catheter

• The inconvenience of caring for the catheter

• The risks of infection or malfunction in the catheter

• The cosmetic effect of an external catheter

HICKMAN CATHETER

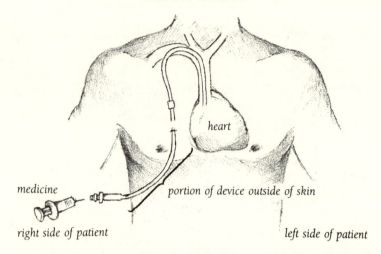

medicine

portion of device outside of skin

right side of patient

left side of patient

Schematic diagram of a Hickman catheter. Medicine, blood, or fluids can be injected into the end of the tube that lies outside of the skin. The rest of the device is under the skin. The catheter ends in or above the right side of the heart.

Many times, even when a problem comes up, there are ways of solving the problem without removing the catheter. Most patients are grateful for the ease and convenience of the catheter.

What Is a Port?

A venous access port is similar to the other central catheters except that the entire device is under the skin. To get blood, or give blood, fluids, or medicines, a needle is inserted through the skin into the implanted chamber. The advantages of ports are:

• They are easier to use and maintain
• They are totally under the skin, and thus are cosmetically preferable

IMPLANTED PORT

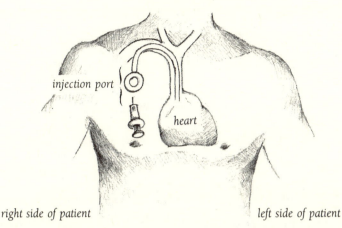

injection port

heart

right side of patient   *left side of patient*

Schematic diagram of an implanted port. The *entire* device is under the
skin. Medicine, blood, or fluids can be injected into the injection port.
Even though the needle goes through the skin into the port, it is a
relatively painless procedure to use this device. There are many
advantages to a totally implantable device.

What Is an Infusion Pump?

A number of portable pumps are now available to deliver a
continuous flow (infusion) of medicine into a vein or artery.
Some therapy is felt to be safer or more effective if given this
way. These are similar to the above-described catheters except
that there is also a device for storing and delivering the medicine under the skin.

How Do I Decide What Treatment to Take?

Weigh and balance the answers to the following questions, and
you will have an idea of what is the best treatment option for
you:

- What are *all* of the treatment options available to me, both conventional and investigational?
- *What are the cure rates of each option?*
- What are the remission rates of each option?
- What are the response rates of each option?
- What are the short-term risks of each option?
    —What is the risk of dying?
    —What are the potential side effects and complications?
- What are the long-term risks of each option?
    —What is the risk of a second cancer?
    —What is the risk of other medical problems?
- Who can provide the treatment?
- Where can I receive treatment?
- How long is each treatment course?
- Will any current treatment limit future treatment options?
- How debilitated will I be from treatment?
    —Will I be able to work?
    —Will I be able to pursue special interests?

If you were basically healthy before your diagnosis of cancer, the key question is: What treatment will give you the best chance?

The right choice is an individual decision. For some people the right choice is treatment with a goal of cure no matter what the chance for cure, or the risks and price of treatment. For others, going for the cure is not the right decision if the chance for cure with treatment is very low, and the price (discomfort, travel, expense, risk of death or complications) is too great.

Doctors can give you numbers regarding each treatment's chance for cure, response, complications, side effects, and death. Doctors and nurses can give some idea of what the experience of treatment will be like. Other patients can give you a closer insight into the experience of treatment. It is valuable to talk to patients who have completed their treatment, as well as patients currently under treatment. Your doctor or nurse can usually refer you to patients who can share with you their experiences and advice.

Do People Ever Stop Their Treatment Before It Is Completed?

If problems come up during your therapy (complications, or poor response of your cancer), you and your physician can re-assess your situation and consider switching to a different therapy. If a newer treatment with clear advantages should become available during your therapy, this can be considered for you, too.

Why Don't I Feel 100 Percent Sure about My Decision Regarding Treatment?

Even with your best efforts, you may feel unsure about your decision regarding treatment. This is because:

- You are being forced to make one of the most important decisions of your life based on statistics and uncertainties. Since no one can give you a guarantee or warranty, there is no way to know for sure that you are making the right decision.
- Unlike taking care of a broken car, which you can re-fix or trade in if the repair does not work, you cannot always re-fix your body and you can never "trade it in for a new one." No other decision you make has this kind of stakes.
- You may be hearing stories of people with similar cancers being treated differently. Everyone and everyone's cancer is

different. You cannot compare yourself with other people unless you know all the details about their situation.

• Lastly, the treatment you choose may involve physical discomforts, time off work or school, significant inconveniences, and emotional stress. You may be fighting fears and worries based on other's stories or past experiences. It is hard to choose something that involves physical and emotional distress.

Take comfort in the knowledge that you are making the best decision at this time. Once you have made your decision, and you have started to proceed, do not look back. devote your energy towards your treatment.

2

Getting into the Medical System

If I Do Not Have an Oncologist (Cancer Specialist),
Do I Need One?

Most people with cancer are treated by an **oncologist**. It can be:

- A medical oncologist—an internist specializing in cancer
- A radiation oncologist—a doctor trained to use radiation to diagnose and treat cancer
- A gynecologic oncologist—a gynecologist specializing in cancer
- A surgical oncologist—a surgeon specializing in cancer

Generally speaking, seeing an oncologist assures that you are getting state-of-the-art treatment by a doctor experienced in the problems special to the cancer patient. Some types of cancer can be treated by an internist or family practitioner. In these cases, it is probably wise to first get an opinion by an oncologist about your treatment.

Do I Need a Second (or Third, or Fourth) Opinion?

If your treatment plan is standard, then a second opinion should be obtained if desired by you and/or required by your insurance company. Deciding what to do about your cancer is such an important decision that many people seek a second opinion even if they have a very common cancer with a very standard treatment.

At least one other opinion is strongly recommended if:

- There are multiple treatment options
- The treatment recommended carries significant risk
- The treatment will affect your life style
- You feel rushed into a decision
- You feel the slightest lack of confidence with the recommended treatment or the doctor

Doctors are here to help you. Doctors expect people to get second and third opinions when people feel they need them. You do not have to worry about a doctor's feelings when you request another opinion.

You can be referred to an oncologist by:

- Your current doctors
- Friends who have been treated for cancer
- Your local medical society
- The American Cancer Society
- The National Cancer Institute's Cancer Information Service (CIS) at 1-800-4-CANCER.

Do I Need To Be Evaluated at a Major Cancer Center?

Well-meaning people may urge you to go to a major cancer center such as M. D. Anderson (Houston) or Memorial Sloan-Kettering Cancer Center (New York). The advantages are:

• Doctors at these centers have considerable experience with all types of cancer, including rare cancers.

• These centers offer investigational programs.

• These centers offer state-of-the-art evaluation and treatment.

The disadvantages are:

• The evaluation can be a less personal experience (you can become a "number").

• It can be expensive, not only in terms of dollars, but in terms of time, travel, and emotional energy.

• It often requires separation from your family and support network.

• A doctor referral is needed (you cannot just go yourself).

Sometimes, local doctors can discuss your case over the phone with doctors at the major centers. As a result, in some cases it is not necessary for you to travel to the cancer center. Your doctor can advise you whether or not a trip is worthwhile.

How Do I Decide If My Doctor Is a Good Doctor for Me?

You can learn about a doctor's credentials by checking the American Medical Directory or the Directory of American Specialists at your local library. If a doctor is Board Certified, he or she passed tests after completing training requirements. Board Certification is one important way to ensure the expertise of the physician.

Factors to consider when choosing a doctor include:

- How experienced is the doctor in your type of cancer and your treatment? You can ask your doctor and/or your doctor's office how many people he or she treats with your situation.
- How well do you communicate with the doctor?
- How comfortable do you feel with the doctor?
- Is the doctor covered by your insurance plan? (You can find this out by asking the doctor's office, or calling the insurance company)
- Where is the doctor's office?
- With what hospital is the doctor affiliated?

You must make your needs clear to the doctor before you decide that a doctor is not right for you. Sometimes it takes a few visits before a good rapport develops. Working with a doctor is a two-way relationship, and in this case a long-term relationship.

Does It Matter with Whom My Doctor "Shares Call"?

Almost all doctors "share call" with other doctors. This means that on weekends, holidays, and possibly weekday evenings, they rotate who is "on call" and therefore who is responsible for patient care. Your doctor is still your primary doctor, but on the days that your doctor is not on call, you can expect to be cared for by the doctor on call should an emergency come up or if you are in the hospital.

Some doctors practice in a "team concept." This means that there is less emphasis on a "primary doctor," and all the doctors share equally in your care. Since having cancer involves a long-term relationship with your doctors, you might consider getting to know the other doctors who will be taking care of you.

Why Does It Matter to What Hospital My Oncologist Admits His or Her Patients?

Even if you are scheduled for all out-patient therapy, there is always the possibility of a hospitalization. This can be to treat a problem

- due to the cancer;
- due to the cancer therapy;
- unrelated to your cancer (e.g., appendicitis).

If you want or need your cancer doctor to be involved, you will have to be admitted to a hospital at which the doctor has admitting privileges. Of course, you can always have other doctors take care of you until you are discharged home, or are well enough to transfer to your cancer doctor's hospital.

Why Do I Have to Put on a Gown at So Many Visits?

Patient gowns serve a very important function: they enable the doctor and nurse to see, hear, and feel as much about your body as possible. Some of your visits will have a physical exam as part of the planned agenda. Other visits will add an examination only after you mention a symptom or problem, or if something comes up on your test results. If you are already in a gown, it is convenient for you, the staff, and the doctor. Being prepared in a gown maximizes the time that is being devoted to evaluating your condition.

Patient gowns are not glamorous or insulated. If you are cold or uncomfortable, ask for a blanket or sweater.

Why Do They Draw Blood at So Many Visits?

Blood tests are an easy way of getting important information about

- your cancer;
- the response of your body to therapy.

Some cancers such as leukemia need close watching to be sure the cancer is not putting you in any new danger. Some treatments, such as chemotherapy, cause changes in your blood that need close monitoring. Changes in your blood can occur over hours to days, so it is common for people to need bloodwork regularly during therapy. Some changes are predictable, others are not. The aim of keeping a close eye on you is to find problems early, when they are easier to treat.

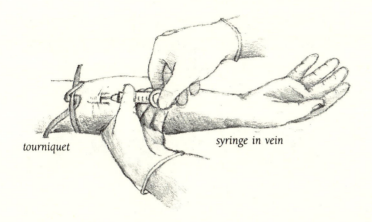

tourniquet   *syringe in vein*

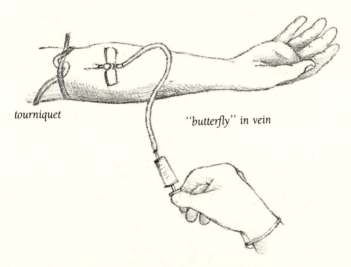

tourniquet   *"butterfly" in vein*

DRAWING BLOOD FOR BLOODTESTS

3

—

Practical Issues

GENERAL MEDICAL CONCERNS

How Should I Proceed If I was Due for a Routine or Followup Exam or Test Unrelated to My Cancer?

Discuss with your doctors whether you should proceed with your routine screening tests or procedures (e.g., stress test, mammogram, colon exam, skin exam, gynecology exam, routine checkup). Some screening tests are part of your cancer workup and need to be done anyway. Also discuss whether your regular doctors or your new doctors should order or do the tests.

Some tests can be safely postponed, and this would allow you to devote your attention to taking care of your cancer. Some tests should not be done at this time, either because they will not give reliable results in the setting of your new illness, or they are unsafe in your current condition. Be sure to discuss your cancer with the doctors who order or perform any tests or procedures before anything is done.

If you have any medical conditions that require routine followup (e.g., high blood pressure, diabetes, heart disease, kidney disease) you should notify your oncologist that you are due for your medical followup. You should also notify your medical doctors that you are being evaluated and treated for cancer (usually they are already aware). Cancer and cancer therapy can affect your medical conditions, and you will need continued followup of these conditions. Sometimes your checkup with your oncologist can replace your checkup with your regular doctor, but usually you will need to continue your routine followups for your medical condition in addition to your visits for your cancer.

Be your own best advocate. Keep up with all of your checkups, cancer-related *and* non-cancer-related. Make sure that each doctor who treats you is aware of what the other doctors are doing. Do not hesitate to ask the doctors to communicate with each other if there are any questions or concerns.

When Should I Call the Doctor?

Medical problems are easier to take care of when they are small or early. A problem taken care of at the inconvenient hour of 2:00 A.M. may be easy to treat. This same problem, if left untreated until the more respectable hour of 8:00 A.M., may end up requiring in-hospital care and be a threat to your life.

In general, *if you feel that something should be brought to the attention of your doctor, call the office or the answering service.* Your doctors do not expect you to be a doctor and know exactly what can wait and what cannot. It is better to have a "false alarm" than have a treatable problem get out of control.

Call your doctor for:

- Fever. Your doctor or nurse will advise you as to what temperature guidelines to use. When blood counts are down, low-grade fevers become very important. Certain cancers cause fevers that do not need to be treated. Make sure you know above what temperature your doctor wants to be notified.
- Shaking chills
- New symptoms or signs (rash, new pain, severe headache, swelling, shortness of breath)
- Inability to keep down fluids or medicines
- Bleeding or bruising
- Increasing pain or uncontrolled pain

Even when you have been forewarned to expect a problem, notify your doctor's office if

- the problem seems worse than you expected;
- the problem is lasting longer than you expected;
- you are quite uncomfortable.

Do I Need Any Vaccinations?

People are more susceptible to infections when they

- have certain cancers;
- are receiving some cancer therapies;
- have had their spleen removed.

Vaccinations are given before a person is exposed to the illness in hopes of building up immunity. Exposure to the infection after a person's immunity is boosted by the vaccination will result in milder illness or no illness.

Vaccines only protect you from the infection covered in the vaccine, and not from all infections. There are some risks involved with vaccinations, and you should discuss with your doctor whether you are a candidate for any vaccinations.

Do I Need a Pneumonia Shot?

The pneumonia shot is a vaccination that helps prevent the most common type of pneumonia, pneumococcal pneumonia. As it takes a few weeks to build up immunity from the vaccination, discuss with your doctor the timing of your vaccination.

The Centers for Disease Control recommends that close contacts (housemates, children, other close associates) of people who need the pneumonia shot also receive the vaccine. This will minimize the chance of a contact bringing the infection to the patient.

Do I Need a Flu Shot?

The flu shot is given every fall (around October) to people at increased risk of influenza. Consider receiving a flu vaccine if you have a serious cancer or will be undergoing therapy that will weaken your immune system.

The Centers for Disease Control recommends that close contacts (housemates, children, other close associates) of people at increased risk for influenza also receive the vaccine.

Do I Need a Hepatitis Vaccine?

The hepatitis vaccine is recommended to people at increased risk of exposure to blood products. It is an expensive three-shot regimen, usually given over six months. There is an optional regimen that can be given over two months. This vaccine may be a consideration depending upon your type of cancer and your proposed treatments.

Can My Children Proceed with Their Routine Vaccinations?

Some vaccinations are "live" vaccines, i.e., they are weakened but alive viruses. If your immune system is weakened by your cancer or will be weakened by your cancer therapy, then exposure to someone who has received a live vaccine may pose a risk to you. Discuss with the children's pediatrician your diagnosis and possible treatments. You will have to balance the children's needs against the risks to you. The pediatrician can tell you which of the children's vaccinations can be safely delayed until your treatment is complete.

Do I Need a Dental Exam?

Yes. A dental exam (cleaning teeth, periodontal work) is recommended prior to starting most chemotherapy or radiation. These cancer treatments can increase the chance of dental problems and/or increase the risk associated with treating any problems that come up during the course of therapy for your cancer.

Make sure that your dentist knows that you are being treated for cancer. If any additional dental work is required during the course of your cancer treatment, discuss it with your cancer doctor before proceeding.

HAIR LOSS

Is Hair Loss Expected?

Radiation can cause hair loss (**alopecia**) at the sites radiated. Some chemotherapy causes hair loss. This is because the treatment works by damaging or killing all the dividing cells that it reaches. Hair loss is temporary in most cases, although high-dose radiation to the scalp can cause permanent hair loss. Hair loss due to chemotherapy affects all body hair, including eyebrows, eyelashes, axillary (armpit) hair, pubic hair, and the hair on your arms and legs.

Your doctor or nurse can advise you as to the likelihood of hair loss or hair thinning with your treatment. They can only give you a likelihood based on experience with the treatments. No one can predict exactly how, if, or when you will lose your hair.

Hair loss can be a traumatic change. It makes you look different than you did before, different from other people, and like a cancer patient.

Try to see your hair loss as a good thing. Hair loss means that your therapy is working on dividing cells in your body. Be reassured by your hair loss that you are also losing cancer cells that are sensitive to the therapy.

If I Do Not Lose My Hair, or My Hair Starts to Grow Back During Therapy, Is the Therapy Still Working on My Cancer?

Yes. There are people whose hair loss is minimal despite use of medicines that usually cause hair loss. It is not uncommon to have hair start to grow back during therapy. These people have the same chance of improvement or recovery from their cancer as people who completely lose their hair.

When Will I Lose My Hair?

If you do lose your hair, you will probably lose it a few weeks after you begin treatment. Some people begin to lose hair a week after their first chemotherapy. How the hair comes out is variable. Your hair may gradually thin out over weeks, or it may fall out in clumps over one to two days.

Should I Order a Wig?

If there is a high likelihood that you will lose your hair, and you think that you will need a wig, it is suggested that you arrange to get a wig before you start losing your hair. The advantages are:

- You can match your hair exactly
- Your wig will be ready for use when you first start to lose hair (or will be ready soon, if custom-made)
- You will have time to practice with it and get it "right" before you really need to wear it
- For some of you, it may be physically easier to go to the wig salon before you start therapy

The disadvantages of getting the wig right away are:

• You may not lose as much hair as expected, and you may not need a wig.

• For some of you, it may be physically easier to go to the wig salon later, if right now you are recovering from surgery or other medical problems.

You can always get fitted for a wig and save the information (style, color, and so on) until after you are sure that you want to order a wig.

Bring one friend or family member with you when you choose your wig. This will make it easier to decide on a wig, as well as help you to remember everything that you are told.

You can find out about reputable wig salons from your oncologist, your nurse, other patients, or your local chapter of the American Cancer Society. There are important differences between "fashion wigs" and "medical wigs" so specify that you need a medical wig.

If you have long hair, it is suggested that you get a short, stylish haircut before you start to lose your hair. The advantages are:

• Long hair that falls out can pull on the remaining long hair, causing clumps.

• It is less dramatic to go from short hair to no hair than from long hair to no hair.

Is a Wig Covered By My Insurance Policy?

Wigs are covered by some insurance policies. Have your oncologist write a prescription for a "cranial prosthesis for alopecia secondary to chemotherapy." Cranial prosthesis is the technical name for a medical wig. Ask your oncologist to avoid writing "hair prosthesis" or "wig" as insurance companies tend to be less enthusiastic about reimbursing when the item is phrased this way. File the prescription with the receipt from the wig salon.

PAIN CONTROL

What Is Causing My Pain?

Pain can be caused by cancer and cancer therapy. It can occur because of

- cancer pressing on something (a nerve, organ, or vessel);
- recent surgery;
- a broken bone;
- a blockage (of a blood vessel, a digestive tube, or the urinary tract);
- skin or bowel changes from radiation;
- mouth irritation from chemotherapy;
- infection;
- swelling.

It is important that you report all pain to your doctor because pain is your body's way of telling you that something is wrong. If you report any new pain (or any new symptom), your doctor can check for a problem or complication that may be easy to treat now, and much harder to take care of later.

The other reason to tell your doctor about any new or persistent pain is to get you relief. There are many safe and effective ways to control pain. Your doctors can offer you options for controlling your pain.

Controlling pain is a team effort. Your doctor can help you only as much as you keep him or her aware of your pain. Your doctor wants to hear about your pain so that something can be done. For many people, it is socially unacceptable to "complain" about pain. This is not a social situation, and reporting pain is not complaining.

There has been so much work done in pain control that there are now "pain control doctors." These doctors work with your regular doctors to get you pain relief if the usual measures do not offer adequate relief.

Remember: Pain can be controlled through a team effort with your doctors. Let your doctors know if you have pain. Let your doctors know if the pain medicine is not working or is causing another problem.

Will I Become Addicted to the Pain Medicine?

Unlikely. Pain medicine that is used to control pain rarely leads to drug addiction. People are able to stop using the pain medicines as soon as the pain is under control.

What If My Family and I Disagree About How Much Pain Medicine I Should Be Taking?

Only you know how much pain you have, and how much your pain is bothering you. Everyone has a different pain threshold. Everyone handles pain medicine differently. You are the one in charge of your pain control. If you feel that you are getting good pain relief, let your family know this. If they still feel that you are "under-medicated," discuss with them why they feel this way. Your nurse and doctor can help you and your family understand how to optimize your pain control.

There are no brownie points given for having pain!

MEDICATION

What Are My Medicines?

Keep a written list of the names and amounts (dosages) of *all* of your medicines because:

- It is easier for you and your doctors to share a written list, especially if you are tired, nervous, or groggy because of medication at the time of your visit.
- A written list minimizes the chance of being given a medicine that you should not get at this time. This is especially true when you see doctors other than your oncologist (e.g., your heart doctor, your dermatologist, your gynecologist).
- If you have to see a doctor who is taking over for your regular doctor (e.g., on a weekend or holiday, or in an emergency), it will be easier and safer for this new doctor to care for you if he/she can see your written list of medications.
- If you get very sick, or have an emergency, the doctor or nurse will want to know the names and amounts of all your medicines. A written list makes it easier for you or someone with you to provide this important information.

Remember: Keep handy a written list of your current medicines. This list should include all prescription and non-prescription medicines. Include anything you are taking for

• your cancer;

• pain control;

• sleep;

• bowel function;

• depression;

• weight loss or gain;

• any medical conditions unrelated to your cancer.

Do I Have to Take All of These Medicines?

Your doctors will assume that you are taking all of your pre-scribed medicines unless you tell them otherwise. Before stop-ping or changing any medicines, discuss it with your doctor. There may be significant danger to stopping a medicine with-out medical supervision.

For some medicines, it is critical that you take them exactly on time (e.g., some chemotherapy, some antibiotics, some pain medicines). The medicines may not work, or they may cause problems, if not taken exactly as directed. Other medicines do not demand such tight control. Find out how important it is to take each medicine on time.

Some medicines are to be taken "as needed" ("**p.r.n.**"). Learn when and how to use these medicines (e.g., some pain medicines, some anti-inflammatories, stool softeners).

How Do I Keep Track of My Medications?

You may be taking more pills than you normally take. Some cancer treatments require a complicated schedule of pill-taking that changes from week to week, or month to month. Taking pills correctly is a big job when you are dealing with emotional stress or you do not feel well.

One way to keep track of your medications is with a "pill-

"PILL-MINDER"

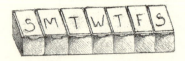

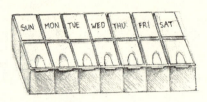

Examples of pill-minders well-suited for medicines taken once a day
(top) and twice a day (bottom).

minder." These are plastic or metal pill boxes that are sold in
pharmacies and grocery stores. Once a week you fill them with
your pills. If you take medication twice a day, it is best to get the
pill-minder that has two slots for each day (for medication
taken three times per day, get the pill-minder with three slots
per day, and so on). If you see pills in your pill-minder, you
will be reminded to take that dose.

Pill-minders are also excellent backup. As long as you are
careful about filling it with the week's medicines, you can simply check your pill-minder to make sure you took your medicine. If by honest error the pharmacy gives you the wrong
number of pills, you will know that you took the right number
of pills because you used your pill-minder.

A second aid that helps keep track of your medications is a
medication list similar to that used in a hospital. Appendix D is
a sample list that you can copy or modify to fit your needs.
Keep the week's list with your medications, and check off each
medication as you take it.

Taking your medicines correctly is an important job. These aids will make the job easier and safer, and thus reduce stress.

NUTRITION

Should I Be On a Special Diet?

Yes. Good nutrition is an important part of your care, and will contribute to your sense of well-being. Nourishment is needed for

- daily functioning (breathing, moving, and so on);
- repair of injured or damaged tissues;
- fighting cancer;
- fighting infection;
- dealing with the body changes due to cancer therapy.

Most people who have cancer or are receiving cancer treatment have an increased need for

- calories;
- protein;
- fluids.

Each person's nutritional needs are unique. Your situation may require special nutritional supplements or dietary restrictions. You can ask for specific guidance from your doctor or nurse. A nutritionist may be involved in your assessment and followup.

Why Do Many People Lose Weight During Treatment for Cancer?

Approximately half of the people with cancer have unintended weight loss due to cancer-induced changes in their body. Some cancers and/or cancer therapy cause one or more of the following:

- decreased appetite;
- decreased taste appreciation;
- nausea;
- trouble swallowing;
- muscle breakdown;
- poor absorption of nutrients from food;
- inefficient use of absorbed nutrients;
- decreased fat storage;
- fasting (e.g. after surgery).

What Can I Do To Avoid Weight Loss?

If you are able to eat, but have a poor appetite, there are many things you can do to make eating easier:

- Think of eating as part of your therapy. Eating well is something that you can do to help yourself get well or feel better.
- Eat what you can eat within any dietary restrictions advised. Do not worry about eating "breakfast foods" at breakfast time, or "lunch foods" at lunch time. If you find a few items that appeal to you, eat them as often as you like. Try to vary your foods as much as possible to avoid getting "burned out" on any particular foods.

- Eat when you can eat; do not worry about eating at "meal times."

- Eat small meals frequently throughout the day. Eat nutritious snacks.

- Discuss food preparation with your nurse or dietician.

- If you do not want to eat solids, or cannot eat solids, try liquid supplements in addition to or in place of meals. Supplements go down fast and easy, and you will be nourishing yourself as if you were eating. These can be bought without a prescription from pharmacies and some grocery stores.

If you are unable to eat, your doctor may discuss nourishing you with tube feedings (liquid feedings through a tube placed into your digestive tract) or intravenous feedings.

If I Was on a Special Diet at the Time of My Diagnosis, Should I Continue It?

If you are on a diabetic, low cholesterol, high calcium, lactose-free, low calorie, or other special diet, discuss with your doctor whether any changes need to be made. Some cancer therapy affects the control of blood sugar or lipids (fats such as cholesterol and triglycerides). Some diets may interfere with your cancer therapy.

Why Does My Diet Seem to Be the Focus of My Family's Attention?

Concern over your diet may cause strain among family members. You may have different ideas than your family does about what to eat, when to eat, or how well you are eating.

For many families, cancer and its treatment is all new, and

difficult to understand. Your diet is something with which family members feel familiar and comfortable. Since your diet is important to your well-being, it becomes one area that they feel they can contribute to your treatment.

Food is also one way people show affection. Concern over your eating habits, and attempts to serve you special foods and meals, are one way that family members try to express love.

Share with your doctor or nurse your family's concerns, preferably with family members present. Clarify what diet you should be on, and whether your current diet is optimal. Communicate to your family exactly how much you do or do not want them involved in your diet. Help family members understand whether their involvement is welcomed for its sense of security as well as practical aid or seen as yet one further loss of independence or sense of self.

Do People Ever Gain Weight While Being Treated for Cancer?

Many people gain weight during therapy for cancer. This can be due to decreased physical activity and/or medications such as steroids. When your cancer is associated with swelling or fluid accumulation, you can gain weight without adding any "fat."

If you have had an overweight problem for a long time, it can be very disappointing to gain weight, especially if you were expecting easy weight loss to be one "good side effect" of having cancer. If you have never had a weight problem, weight gain can be distressing. Ways to combat weight gain include:

• Limit "empty" calories (e.g., potato chips, candy, and so on).

• Stay as active as your medical condition allows.

If I Am Overweight, Can I Try to Lose Weight?

In most cases, this is not the time to try to lose weight. Weight loss due to cancer or poor intake of food is not a healthy weight loss. Dieting to lose weight may deprive your body of the fuel it needs to fight the cancer or deal with the treatments.

Is There a Special Diet to Prevent Cancer?

The American Cancer Society recommends a set of dietary guidelines to help decrease the risk of developing cancer. *These recommendations are* not *to be followed when you are diagnosed with cancer, or are recovering from a course of cancer treatment. The cancer prevention diet could interfere with your body's ability to fight your cancer or recover from your therapy.*

If you have never had cancer or you are completely recovered from cancer therapy, the American Cancer Society recommends that you:

- Avoid obesity
- Eat a low-fat diet
- Eat dietary fiber
- Eat cruciferous vegetables (cabbage, broccoli, brussels sprouts, cauliflower)
- Avoid excessive alcohol consumption
- Be moderate in consumption of salt-cured, smoked, and nitrite-cured foods

WORK AND SCHOOL

Will I Be Able to Continue Working or Studying While I Undergo Testing?

Discuss with your doctor and your family how you should handle your immediate work or school situation. Sometimes your medical situation leaves you little choice but to take at least a short leave of absence. Even if you feel well, adjusting to a diagnosis of cancer is a major stress. Many people need some time just to gather themselves and take care of immediate issues (dealing with family, doctor's appointments, taking care of insurance, getting a wig).

Short-term leave may be needed for:

• Recuperation from surgery or procedures
• Emotional adjustment
• Completion of your evaluation
• Beginning treatment

Will I Be Able to Continue Working or Studying While I Undergo Treatment?

Many people work or study full-time or part-time during cancer therapy. Whether you can work or continue school will depend on:

• How rigorous your treatment is
• How rigorous your treatment schedule is

- How flexible your job or school is about schedule
- How demanding your job or school is, physically and emotionally
- How well you are doing physically
- How well you are doing emotionally

Long-term leave may be needed if:

- Treatment may make you unable to perform your usual duties;
- Your work may put you at risk during treatment (e.g., a nurse exposed to sick kids all day would be at risk for serious infection while undergoing some chemotherapy treatments).

Do I Have to Tell My Boss about My Cancer Diagnosis? Should I Tell My Colleagues, Coworkers, Subordinates, Students, and So on, about My Cancer Diagnosis?

How much you tell will depend on your particular work situation, your personal situation, and your personality.

The advantages of sharing your news are:

- There will be no misunderstanding about why you look or act different than usual (speculation can be worse than the truth)
- You will not have to put up quite as convincing a "front" on difficult days
- You will not have to create excuses or explanations when you need to make schedule changes or if people notice any changes in you

• You may find an important support system at work

The disadvantages of sharing your news are:

• You may have to deal with other people's fears, concerns, and prejudices about your situation;

• You may have to deal with people's sympathetic concern for you on days that you feel great and would just like to forget that you have or had cancer. ("How are you doing today? When is your next checkup?");

• You may be disappointed by some people's lack of concern or lack of sympathy when you need it.

All states provide legal protection from discrimination due to a handicap. Much attention has been focused on the rights of cancer patients, and whether having cancer or having a history of cancer makes a person "handicapped." An individual's legal protection in this regard varies from state to state.

INSURANCE

How Do I Start Dealing with the Insurance Company?

• *Make sure your premiums are up to date!*

• Obtain a copy of the most current plan booklet from your insurance carrier.

• Obtain some blank insurance claim forms.

• Make a copy of everything that you submit for payment.

- Make a copy of all communications to insurance companies.

- Keep the Explanation of Benefits form ("EOB") together with your copy of the claim form and invoice.

- Review your bills for accuracy; review what has been paid by your insurance company. Errors do occur.

- Submit claims for everything for which you are billed, including wigs and medications.

- If a claim is denied, and you feel that this is in error, then have the doctor's office and the insurance company advise you how to pursue reimbursement.

- Check to see if you have a "waiver of premium" feature (i.e., the policy that you purchased provides for no premiums to be paid during the time of illness or disability).

- Your doctors' offices and the insurance company can help advise you which bills will probably be covered by your insurance.

Obtaining new insurance after you have been diagnosed with cancer is becoming very difficult and expensive. It is very important that you keep your policies in force by paying all required premiums on time and in full. Attention to your policy is now a top priority.

Am I Going to Be Able to Get Insurance If I Switch Jobs?

There are cases of people feeling "locked in" to their current jobs after a diagnosis of cancer because of problems getting insurance if they switch jobs. Whether or not you can get insurance depends upon the specific insurance policy. With some policies, it makes a difference what type of cancer you have or had.

Laws are changing regarding insurability. There is a strong lobbying effort being made by cancer survivors and survivors of other major illnesses to make it easier to get insurance.

Is There Anything That I Can Do If My Claim Is Denied?

Yes! If your insurance company denies payment on a claim, do not give up. Be persistent. Find out from the insurance company why it was rejected. Resubmit the claim. Have your doctor's office help you if you feel a legitimate claim was denied. In a large, bureaucratic organization such as an insurance company, "the squeaky wheel gets the grease."

Is There Anyone Who Can Do My Insurance Filing for Me?

Most major cities have professional claim-filing services that you can hire to file your bills. They are listed in the Yellow Pages under "insurance claim-processing services." Some of these services are for physicians only. Some of the major insurance companies have a service available whereby one of their carrier representatives will file for a patient and/or work with the patient on their medical claims.

WILLS / LIVING WILLS

Do I Need to Do Anything About My Will?

Everyone needs a will, whether they have cancer or not. You are urged to make sure that your will is up to date. Also make sure that family, friends, or your physician knows where your will is kept. If you do not have a will, it is suggested that you obtain a lawyer and do it now if:

- You are very ill
- You are going to have high-risk surgery or a high-risk procedure
- You are not very ill, and you feel that you can handle it emotionally

Do I Really Need to Think about a Will Right Now?

Tending to your will does not mean in any way that you are going to die soon, or that you think that you might die soon. Simply put, we all should have wills at all times so that if anything should happen to us (e.g., car accident, fatal heart attack), those left behind would handle our affairs the way we would like. A well-written will minimizes problems for those tending to our affairs, and decreases the amount lost to taxes.

A will is a sensitive issue to discuss, especially if you have just been diagnosed with cancer. If you are struggling with your new diagnosis, then it may be difficult and damaging to bring up the emotionally charged issue of a will. If you are unsure whether you or your family can handle a discussion of your will, have your doctor or a hospital social worker give you and your family some guidance on how to deal with this matter.

What Is a Living Will?

A **living will** is a written statement that outlines what you would or would not like done to prolong your life artificially should recovery become almost impossible. This document can be written when a person is totally healthy, or after an illness has occurred. You must be considered able (competent) to sign a living will. There is an active movement underway to encourage people to get living wills because you never know if you are going to be in an accident or have an unexpected medical emergency.

What Is the Patient Self-Determination Act?

On December 1, 1991, the Patient Self-Determination Act went into effect, which requires hospitals, nursing facilities, hospices, home health care programs, and health maintenance organizations to:

- give adults information about their rights under state law to accept or refuse treatment;
- help the patient prepare a living will or appoint a medical proxy if they wish to do so.

What Is Durable Power of Attorney?

Durable power of attorney is a legal document that allows the person you specify in the document to make health care decisions for you in the event that you are unable to do so. The person you specify is called your "proxy" or "health care agent."

Who Will Make My Health Care Decisions if I Am Unable, and I Have Not Prepared a Living Will or Durable Power of Attorney?

If you are unable to make decisions and you have not prepared a living will or assigned a health care proxy, the decision to continue or end your treatment will be made by your physician and family. In some cases, the hospital will become involved. If there is controversy, the court can become involved.

An example of a living will is included in Appendix G. You can obtain more information and/or a blank form from your doctor, your lawyer, or:

Society for the Right to Die
250 West 57th Street
New York, N.Y. 10107

4

The Emotional Adjustment

FEELINGS

How Am I Supposed to Feel?

There is no right way to feel after you have been told you have cancer. Whatever you feel is the right way for you. Common, normal feelings and reactions include

- Fear
- Confusion
- Anger
- Panic
- Loneliness
- Sadness, grief

- Sense of unreality
- Crying
- Irrational thoughts
- Change in appetite
- Change in sleeping pattern, including nightmares
- Diminished or absent sexual drive
- Sense of loss of control
- Difficulty making decisions
- Irritability
- Poor concentration

You may have none, some, or all of these feelings and reactions. The feelings may be vague and mild, or very extreme. They can come and go. These reactions are your body's way of adjusting to the new situation. Some of these feelings can be due to your medications.

Let your feelings and reactions happen. Talk about them with friends, family, your nurse, a support group, or someone else who has been through a similar experience. Write about your reactions and feelings in a diary or a letter. Professional counseling may be enormously beneficial, enabling you to get through this initial phase more quickly and with less emotional distress than if you worked through your feelings on your own. Counseling is available from nurse therapists, clinical social workers, psychologists, psychiatrists, and clergypersons.

You will not feel like this forever; these feelings will lessen with time. Be sure that you continue to get medical attention during this adjustment phase. You cannot let your emotions interfere with your getting proper care for your cancer.

Being told you have cancer is a major event in your life. **What thoughts and feelings you have are not as important as what you do with them.**

How Do I Know If I Need a Therapist?

You do not have to be emotionally unstable to benefit from counseling. Many people who have been emotionally healthy their entire lives and who are reacting "normally" to their new cancer diagnosis benefit from the interaction with a professional counselor. You can shorten the time of adjustment, and make the transition easier, with counseling. Do not hesitate to have your oncologist refer you to a trained therapist if you are feeling overwhelmed, afraid, anxious, depressed, or if you are having difficulty concentrating, relating to others, or fulfilling your responsibilities.

Athletes work with counselors, training their emotions and concentration in order to improve their athletic performance. Dealing with cancer is a challenge that demands energy for physical healing. Do not spend weeks or months wasting precious energy dealing with difficult emotions and thoughts. Just as well-adjusted athletes benefit from counseling, well-adjusted cancer patients benefit from counseling.

Why Am I Having Trouble Believing That This is Really Happening?

It is common for people with a new diagnosis of cancer to say, "I cannot believe that this is happening" or "I feel like this is all a bad dream and I am going to wake up."

This is the numbing effect of the shock. Numbness protects us from the initial trauma and is normal. This reaction can last days or even months. If it lasts longer than that, you will need some help to move on with your adjustment.

Even if you are experiencing numbness or disbelief, you must still proceed with getting attention to your cancer. If you cannot make decisions or bring yourself to get medical attention, have your doctor direct you to people or support groups who can help you through this early phase. Even if you are able to fulfill your responsibilities, if your feelings seem overwhelming let your doctors connect you with people who will help you through this adjustment phase.

Having trouble believing this is really happening is normal. Denying that this is happening is not normal, and heals nobody.

Why Me?

This is a question commonly asked, often repeatedly, by people who are told they have cancer. This is a deep question that touches on your beliefs about life and God.

It is a fact of the human condition that life involves pain, loss, and death. You are human; you cannot escape the human condition.

When cancer is diagnosed, even well-adjusted, mature people can find themselves with thoughts such as, "If this bad thing is happening to me, then I must have been bad." This is a common, human, natural reaction for many people. Thinking about "why me?" can make you feel guilty, angry, overwhelmed, helpless, or isolated. Friends, family, ministers or rabbis, and counselors can help you deal with this question later on.

Right now, the practical and useful question is not "Why me?" but "What can I do about my situation now?"

How Should I Feel If Something I Did May Have Caused the Cancer or Allowed It to Get as Far as It Did?

If you did something in the past that may have contributed to your current cancer situation, such as smoked cigarettes or delayed a mammogram, it is understandable that you may feel guilty. Chances are you down-played, denied, or did not know the risks of your behavior to yourself before you were diagnosed with cancer. Guilt is good when it helps you to do the right thing, not when you beat yourself up with it. Focusing on what you should have done, or could have done, is destructive, wasted energy. Blaming yourself helps no one, and hurts you. You did not want to get cancer. Forgive yourself for being human and imperfect.

Is Denial a Good Thing?

Technically speaking, denial is an abnormal refusal to accept the truth. In this book, the word denial will be used loosely, as it is by most non-psychiatrists, to mean anything from unhealthy denial of the truth to healthy repression of painful truths.

There is a place for healthy denial in life. We use denial every day. If we thought about everything bad that could happen every time we drove on the highway, or let our children ride their bicycles, we would be stuck in a world that was filled with fear, anxiety, and immobility. It is healthy and normal to use some denial, as long as we are responsible in our behavior.

Right now, you may be imagining all the possible bad things that could happen from your cancer or your cancer therapy. You have temporarily lost your ability for healthy denial. This will change. If it does not improve with time, you can get help to regain your healthy ability to deny.

If you deny that you have cancer, or deny symptoms or problems, you are risking your health and your life. This kind of denial is not good.

SHARING THE DIAGNOSIS

Who Should I Tell about My Cancer?

This is a personal issue. It depends upon your social circumstances, the relationships you have, and your personality. If you tend to share, and have people with whom you can share, then you will probably get much-needed support by sharing your news. If you tend to be very private and independent, then you will probably involve the minimum number of people in your new situation.

Should I Tell the Children?

Yes. Children will sense that something is going on. In general, it is best to be open and honest with children, *on their level*. What they can understand will depend upon their age and maturity. If you do not say anything, their imagination may bring them to conclusions and fears that are much worse than the real situation. Listen to the children. Let them guide you as to how much they want to know. If they ask questions, answer them as simply as possible. Children are affected by *how* you answer as much as by *what* you actually say.

Your children's pediatrician and teachers can give you some specific guidance about how best to deal with your children (or children with whom you associate). Do not wait for a problem to seek the input and involvement of your children's pediatrician and teachers.

- *Tell the children that you have cancer, and that you are going to be treated.* It is much better to tell them yourself than risk their overhearing it in your conversations with others, or hearing it for the first time from someone else. If they hear it from you, they know that they can trust you to tell them the truth about what is going on.

- *Make it clear that cancer is not contagious.* They cannot get cancer from you if they are close to you. They did not give the cancer to you.

- *Make it clear that cancer is a disease, and not a death sentence.* Children can have preconceptions about cancer from television, friends' comments, or their interpretation of what is happening around them. If it is expected that you will do well, you need to say this directly. If you are not expected to do well, you need to make it clear that this is because of your particular situation and not just because you have cancer.

- *Tell the children that they did not cause your cancer.* Do not assume that the children know this. Depending upon their age, children can believe that you got cancer because they did something "bad," or even just thought something "bad." You may need to reinforce this over and over.

- *Children, including teenagers, need reassurance that their needs will be satisfied.* It is normal and healthy for children to be anxious and/or angry about what is going to happen to them. As upsetting and demanding as your situation may seem to you, you must remember that this crisis is affecting the children close to you. If you cannot tend to their needs, ask someone else to be there for their physical and emotional needs. You may save yourself and the children from future problems by being responsive to their needs now.

GETTING HELP

Why Should I Ask for Help?

You may be experiencing:

- Emotional stress
- Additional time demands of your evaluation and treatment
- Physical stress from tests or surgeries

Accepting help has many advantages:

- You can devote your time and energy to taking care of your medical needs, and the decisions ahead of you.
- You can get more rest, if you want or need it.
- You will have more time to communicate with your family and friends, create a support network, and work out some of your feelings.

Family and friends want to help you. The only way they can help is by doing errands, making meals, talking, and listening. By asking people for help, you are offering them an opportunity to enrich their lives.

You help yourself and help others by accepting help.

What Kind of Help Do I Need?

The kind of help you need will depend on your circumstances. You may need help with:

- Meals
- Transporting you to appointments
- Babysitting
- Transporting children to school, activities, or doctor appointments
- Housekeeping
- Shopping (food, house supplies, gifts)
- Unexpected problems (broken car, leaking freezer, and so on)

Depending upon your past experience with cancer, other people may be able to help you by:

- Getting information about your cancer, and your treatment
- Being a "reader," someone who can read the information provided to you, and research any additional information
- Being a "listener," someone who can accompany you to your appointments and listen to all the questions and answers
- Finding out about home health care, if needed

How Do I Ask for Help?

Many people feel uncomfortable asking for help. Having cancer is not "usual circumstances," and it is a most appropriate time to ask for help.

When people call to offer something that is on your "need" list, say "yes," and allow them to fulfill that need. If they call to offer general help, tell them your list of needs and see if they can help out in any of these areas. If they cannot help at this time, tell them that their concern is appreciated, and that you will contact them should any new needs arise.

You do not owe it to anyone to tell them the details of your medical situation. If you want them to know, but do not want to go through the story yourself, you can have someone else do the calling and explaining. If you do not want them to know the specifics, you are entitled to be vague: "I have some important appointments that I cannot reschedule," "I am going through some hard times that I cannot talk about right now," "I am having some medical problems, but I do not want to talk about them yet."

Depending on your medical and personal situations, you may need help for a long time, maybe months. Let people know how long you think you might need help. Otherwise, people could disappear from the helping scene because they are unaware that your need still exists.

There are many people who want to help and are able to help. Give them the opportunity to help by making your needs known.

Where Do I Ask for Help?

Family and close friends are usually aware of your situation, and will let you know if they can help. If you are part of a religious congregation, let them know your situation. You may find yourself with offers from casual acquaintances and even strangers from your congregation. Social or athletic organizations may have members who are able to help.

If you do not have access to family, friends, neighbors, a religious community or other social community, there are many local and national volunteer support groups that provide information and hands-on help. Doctors, nurses, and hospital social workers are familiar with organizations that provide service.

What Is A Support Group?

Generally speaking, a support group is any person or people who are willing and able to help you, emotionally or physically. A "support group" may also refer to an organized group that meets regularly to deal with cancer-related issues. There are cancer support groups where people with any type of cancer get together to deal with issues common to all cancer patients. There are also support groups that are geared towards people with specific cancers or specific problems.

Do I Need to Participate in a Support Group?

Everyone who is physically able should try participating in a support group. Find out which support groups are available from your local hospital's social work department or the local office of the American Cancer Society. Support groups can:

• Be a good way to get practical information

• Provide a support network separate from family, coworkers, and past friends. This is especially helpful for people who have chosen to minimize the involvement of their established relationships.

• Provide a support network of people who truly understand because they have been cancer patients, too.

• Provide exposure to people who have chosen to make a good life despite their cancer or cancer history.

Support groups are not for everyone. The quality of each support group varies depending upon the theme, the leaders, and the individuals who participate. People can find it frightening or upsetting to see other people who are worse off than they are, or listen to someone who has a negative attitude or a depressing personality. The only way to know if a support group will be beneficial to you or your family is to try one.

How Do I Find Out about the Support Groups Available to Me?

You can find out about local support groups by calling:

- Your local chapter of the American Cancer Society
- Your local hospital's social service department
- Your oncologist's office
- The National Coalition for Cancer Survivorship (NCCS) (301) 585-2616

How Do I Deal with People Who Seem Uncomfortable Dealing with Me?

Unfortunately, some people do feel uncomfortable dealing with someone else's hard times, especially illness. It may be that they genuinely want to help, but do not know how. For these people, the simplest thing to do is to be direct:

Thanks for calling [or writing]. This is all new to me, and I appreciate your concern. I would like to share some thoughts with you . . .

. . . I am not ready to talk, but could you call again in a week or two? Can I call you?

. . . I get plenty of support from my family and my support group, but I would really like to go for a walk and talk about things other than cancer.

Some "friends" do disappear in the face of illness, even if you make it easy for them to keep contact. This can make you feel sad, insecure, angry, or lonely. You may feel as if you did something wrong. These people may have their own hangups about illness. You need to see this as their problem, not yours. Since you have lost a friend, and lost an image of this friend, you will likely experience some grief. Try as best as you can to focus on the important tasks at hand, and not on the disappointing response of some people.

I Feel Uncomfortable Saying the Word "Cancer." What Should I Do?

"Cancer" is a very emotional word for some people. It is common to have difficulty saying the word cancer because of all the frightening things that you associate with cancer.

The right way to handle this is whatever feels comfortable for you. Find the word or phrase that you find the easiest to say now ("tumor," "malignancy," "problem"). Do what is comfortable for you, not for other people. If you are not ready to use the word cancer yet, don't.

Many people with cancer find that the more they use the word cancer, the less and less emotional or scary it becomes. Cancer becomes just one more regular word in your vocabulary. Other people may be offended or uncomfortable if you use the word cancer frequently. That is their problem, not yours.

FAMILY CONCERNS

Some Family Members Have Become Worried about Getting Cancer Themselves. Is This Normal?

It is understandable that people close to you may become more conscious of any symptoms they may have, or simply become worried that they, too, will develop cancer. After all, if you could get cancer, then they could.

If the person has any symptoms, it is best to get them checked out now by a doctor. If there is a problem, it will be tended to. If there is not a problem, the reassurance will relieve the person and you.

What about Sex?

It is common for people's interest in sex to diminish or disappear after they are first diagnosed with cancer. Sexual desire and sexual function can be affected by

- Stress
- Anxiety
- Depression
- Fatigue
- Physical problems or changes
- Medications
- Some treatments

There are volumes written about the effects of cancer and treatment on sexual function and sexual satisfaction. Doctors, nurses, counselors, and support groups are all trained to guide you through this transition. If you have questions, concerns, anxieties, or problems, let your doctor know. Doctors consider your sexuality a part of your normal functioning, just like your eating, sleeping, and breathing. By discussing questions or problems you can decrease the chance of

• unnecessary restrictions and limitations;

• future problems.

Whereas sexual desire may be diminished, your need for intimacy may be increased. Being close, hugging, and talking privately are important ways to combat loneliness and isolation. It is important for you and for those who care about you to maintain contact.

Why Are Things So Strained with Some of My Family?

Even under ideal circumstances, being diagnosed with cancer causes strain in family relationships. This is because you and your family are dealing with fears, changes in roles and responsibilities, and oftentimes fatigue.

Those relationships that were less than ideal before your diagnosis will also be under strain. Many times, people "rise to the occasion" and you finally smooth out a rocky or unstable relationship. Other times, the relationship just gets worse under the added stress. This is an especially difficult time for you to deal with family problems, more stress, or more loss. If you are having problems with your family, ask your doctor, your nurse, or a social worker to help you deal with these issues. These professionals are trained to deal with family problems, and can give you the best chance of dealing with them in a healthy, productive way.

THE MIND-BODY CONNECTION

What Is a "Cancer Personality"?

In your readings or discussions, you may come across the idea of a "cancer personality"—a type of person who is more likely to get cancer because of his or her personality. There is no rigorous, scientific study to support the concept of a cancer personality. All different types of people do get cancer. There are millions of people with the supposed cancer personality who do not get cancer. You did not cause your cancer. Your personality did not cause your cancer.

It is interesting to look back in history at explanations for illnesses that are now well-defined. For example, before the organism that causes tuberculosis was discovered, people hypothesized about a "tuberculosis personality."

Is There Any Truth in All the Talk about Curing Ourselves with Better Stress Management and a Positive Outlook?

There is much work being done on the relationship of emotions, attitudes, and coping styles to the chance of survival after cancer has developed. Improving your chances with healthy stress management and a positive outlook is not a new concept, and it is accepted as truth by most lay and professional people. If done in a way that fits your personality and preferred life style, stress management and an optimistic outlook at the very least will make you feel better.

The new twist is that some books, articles, and talk shows leave you with the impression that if you do not learn to manage all your stress and if you do not always have an optimistic outlook, then you are hurting your chances for improvement or cure. This approach leads to guilt and more stress. Normal life carries stress, pain, loss, and worries. If you try to protect yourself from these things, then you will be isolating yourself physically and emotionally from your real life. Trying to avoid life's stresses can cause more stress than the original stress!

A positive attitude and improved stress management will be an important part of your recovery, but these things take time.

Self-help books prescribe attitudes, diets, and rituals that are very helpful for some people. For others this well-intentioned advice causes problems: if the person dismisses the advice because he or she does not believe in it, there may be some guilt about not doing "everything possible." Strain can arise from people with cancer rejecting, or following only half-heartedly, the advice of friends and loved ones about a particular diet or ritual (e.g., meditation).

There is definitely a place for looking at your life style and attitude and deciding to change some things about the way you live your life. You do not have to change anything right now. You will have a better idea of what you want to change when the initial phase of adjustment and treatment is over.

The right attitude and right level of stress is whatever is best for you. Open your eyes to different outlooks, approaches, and styles. Try out ideas that may work for you. Reject ideas that are not for you. Many people use this situation as an opportunity to change things for the better.

What about Hypnosis?

Hypnosis can be a safe and effective way to help control pain, nausea, anxiety, or other unpleasant side effects of cancer and cancer therapy. Professionals trained in hypnosis teach you to achieve a state of relaxed consciousness such that your subconscious is more susceptible to helpful suggestion (i.e., "I will be hungry for lunch after I finish today's chemotherapy," "I will be calm when I go for my CAT scan"). With time, patients learn to achieve this state on their own (self-hypnosis). Hypnosis can be thought of as an extension of self-relaxation, biofeedback, visual imagery, or meditation.

People can be reluctant to consider hypnosis because of their image of a magician using hypnosis to levitate a subject. In modern, practical terms, hypnosis is a simple technique that enables you to have more control over your body's functions. Make sure that the hypnotist, oftentimes a psychiatrist, is well-trained in this skill.

5

Insights and Handles for Getting You Through

What Can I Do to Make Life Easier These Next Few Months?

Millions of people have traveled this cancer journey before you. The experience of these veterans provides insights and handles for helping you through. There is no way to eliminate all the emotions, discomforts, inconveniences, worries, strain, and uncertainties.

You can learn ways to cope with the difficulties of having cancer. You can learn tricks and philosophies that will make the hard times easier.

The following thoughts may explain some of what is happening in your life right now, and give you the tools you need to travel this unexpected journey:

EXPECT STRONG EMOTIONS AND REACTIONS

Your reactions and emotions are real, no matter how extreme. For normal, healthy people this is a very difficult situation. Chances are that you are not overreacting and that you are handling it as well as can be expected. Do not hesitate to have your doctor get you in touch with someone who can help determine if you would benefit from counseling.

CANCER IS A FAMILY AFFAIR

The diagnosis of cancer affects everyone who is close to you. There are the practical effects as you may be unable to fulfill your usual responsibilities and others have to assume these tasks. There are the emotional effects as people around you deal with their own shock, fears, anxieties, and grief brought on by learning that you have cancer. As difficult as this situation may be for you, remember that it is difficult for those who care for you.

FOCUS ON WHAT YOU CAN DO NOW TO HELP YOUR SITUATION

Regretting or worrying about the past is a waste. You cannot change the past so do not spend time, energy, or emotion looking back at what you did, what you did not do, and what you could have done. If you find yourself thinking about the past, tell yourself to focus on what you can do now.

THE ''ROLLER-COASTER'' OF CANCER

Dealing with cancer is like being on a roller-coaster. You will have days when you feel you can handle it, and then days when you feel it is overwhelming. The checkups, tests, treatment-related problems, and uncertainty and changes in your daily life cause fluctuating anxiety, depression, frustration, and disappointment. When you are having a "good" day, enjoy it! When you are having a "bad" day, remember that it is okay to have a bad day, and that tomorrow may be better.

THE LOSS OF CONTROL

Having cancer makes you painfully aware of how little control you now have over many important things. You get test results that you cannot change. You have to deal with anxiety-producing and time-consuming medical appointments, treatments, and discomforts.

We all try to control our lives to some degree. Lack of control makes people anxious, frustrated, or angry. The truth of the matter is that we cannot completely control our lives, including our health. Even when you do everything "right," bad things happen (accidents, robberies, cancer). When you accept this lack of control as a fact of life, you are free to focus your energy on the things that you can control.

SAY "NO" TO THINGS THAT ARE NOT HELPING

You do have some control over the things to which you are being exposed. Control things that are not good for you. If a news show or movie is upsetting you, turn it off. If someone's conversation is upsetting you, tell them that it is not a good conversation for you right now, or leave. These actions do not mean that you are weak. These actions show that you are strong enough to recognize what is not good for you now. You are preserving your emotional well-being. Listen to yourself to know what is good for you and what is not good for you now.

LEARN TO CONTROL BAD THOUGHTS OR EXPERIENCES

Find little thoughts or phrases that help you handle the inconveniences, discomforts, fears, and disappointments of dealing with cancer. Everyone is different, and you will have to find the "handles" that work for you.

Some examples:

• When you have to undergo needle sticks, or other uncomfortable procedures, instead of thinking about how much you have to "suffer," think of it as something you have to "put up with."

• When you go for a treatment, think of it as one treatment closer to being better.

• When you see unpleasant changes due to your treatment (e.g., hair loss), think of these as signs that the treatment is doing its job.

• Think of your treatment as "the way for me to get some relief or get cured," "something good for me," "my friend." Do not think of your treatment as "nasty" or "bad."

• If you have pain or a problem now, deal with it as it is now, and do not start worrying about how it might be worse tomorrow. Worrying about tomorrow may make today's pain seem worse, and will not help you deal with tomorrow when tomorrow comes.

GRIEVING FOR YOUR LOSSES

Having cancer involves a lot of losses: the loss of health, the loss of work or school, the possible loss of future plans or dreams, the loss of hair, and the loss of illusion that you are safe from injury, illness, or death. The human reaction to loss is grieving. You can expect to grieve for all the big and little losses over the next few weeks to months.

YOUR LIFE WILL NEVER BE THE WAY IT WAS

Once you have cancer, your life will never be the same. It can be difficult to accept change, especially this unexpected, un-desired kind of change. Remember that all of life is about change: learning to walk means giving up complete depen-dence, having children means taking on responsibilities and limitations, choosing one career means not pursuing another, being alive means growing older. You are still the same person, just taking one of the sharper "bends" in your life.

LAUGH A LITTLE!

You do not have to be sad or serious all the time. In fact, there is good evidence to indicate a comforting and healing effect of laughter and happiness. It is healthy to let yourself forget about your situation. Try to escape any way you can—a movie, candid-camera videos, comic books, going to a party. Let the people around you know that it is okay for you to be happy when you can.

FIND THE BEST COPING METHOD FOR YOU

There are as many different ways to cope as there are people. You are a unique individual, and you will find the best coping style for you. If something has worked well for you in the past, it will probably help you now. This can also be a time to learn new ways of coping. You may try one way, find it just does not work for you, and then try another. One coping tool may work well now, and not later. Another may not work right now, but will work fine later.

Some places that can guide you with coping methods include

- Religious groups
- Cancer support groups
- Self-help books
- Counseling
- Discussion with a cancer "survivor"

(See Appendix C)

SET GOALS

Set goals for yourself every day. Think of something that you want to get done, or need to get done. The goals can be as little as making a phone call, writing a letter, reading the newspaper, or making lunch. If you are able, focus on bigger projects, too.

Make the goals reasonable. When you accomplish a goal, enjoy the satisfaction of a job done.

BE A ''GOOD'' PATIENT

Your doctor is trying to solve your little and big problems with sensitivity and efficiency. If you make it easier for him or her, your doctor can do a better job for you.

Some hints for being a "good" patient include:

- Come prepared for your visits with a list of the most important issues that should be discussed.

- If you know that you will need extra time at a visit, let the person who does the scheduling set aside time for a longer visit, so that your doctor is not rushed by other commitments.

- Be honest about your symptoms or problems. The more clues your doctor has, the better chance there is of determining what the problem is, and getting it taken care of. Withholding information because you "do not want to complain" or "do not want to take up the doctor's time" or "think it is not important enough" may end up being very expensive for you in terms of delayed diagnosis, extra tests, and delayed treatment.

- If you are unsure about the importance of a symptom, let the doctor or nurse decide if it needs attention. They will let you know if something needs to be done. With time, you will learn what to call for, and what can wait for the next visit. It is better to be safe than sorry.

- Tell your doctor if you or your family have emotional or social questions or concerns. These things affect your medical condition. If your doctor cannot tend to them personally, he or she can get you the assistance you need. At the very least, it is best for you and your doctor if he or she is aware of your situation.

- Tell your doctor if you have a problem with something he or she, or the staff, is doing. Give specific examples.
- Tell your doctors how much information you want them to share with your family.
- Leave the office only after you are clear about
  1. Your next appointment
  2. Your instructions
  3. Your prescriptions
  4. What you should call the office for
- Know when you are due for your appointments, tests, treatments, or followup calls. Do not depend on the office or hospital to remind you when you are to come in. If you think you are supposed to be scheduled for a test, and the office has not scheduled it, or seems to know nothing about it, ask them to check with the doctor. Do not assume that the test was canceled, or that you were in error.

Conclusion

You are a cancer patient. You did not choose to be a cancer patient. Right now, not having cancer is not an option. The good thing is that you are a cancer patient with choices—choices about your evaluation, your treatment, how you spend your time, how you relate to other people, how you see your situation, and how you cope. My hope is that *Diagnosis: Cancer Your Guide Through the First Few Months* has helped you to see your choices and take the best choices for you.

The first few months after a diagnosis of cancer are a transition period for you. For most people, it is unsettling to deal with all the physical, social, and emotional changes of having cancer. My hope is that this book has made it easier by showing you some tricks of passage.

Diagnosis: Cancer Your Guide Through the First Few Months is just a start. The bibliography in Appendix B offers suggestions of books that are helpful resources for coping with all aspects of the cancer experience. The resource list in Appendix C directs you to support groups and individuals who can help you with everything from insurance forms to dealing with the emotional stress of having cancer.

Having cancer is a very personal experience. Everyone comes into the experience a unique individual. Everyone finds their own unique way of handling the experience. Having cancer is not easy. Learning about cancer and about how to cope with cancer can make it much easier. Having cancer is not good. Learning about cancer and about how to cope with cancer can enable you to feel that some good things can come out of this situation.

As they say in baseball, you can't choose your pitches, but you can choose how you hit the ball.

As they say in poker, you can't choose your hand, but you can choose how you play it.

Glossary

Abdomen: Part of the body below the diaphragm; contains the stomach, kidneys, pancreas, intestines, and other organs.

Adenocarcinoma: Cancer that started in glandular tissue (e.g., breast, lung, thyroid, colon, pancreas).

Adjuvant chemotherapy: Chemotherapy given when there is no evidence by any tests for leftover cancer but there is reason to be concerned that there are still cancer cells in the body. It is given with the expectation of decreasing the chance of a recurrence.

Alopecia: Hair loss.

Anaplastic: A cancer whose cells, under the microscope, look very immature and different from the tissue in which it started. Sometimes it is impossible to be sure where it started. These are usually faster-growing cancers.

Anemia: "Low blood count," low red blood cells or hemoglobin, due to blood loss, blood destruction in the vessels, or impaired ability to make new blood.

Angiogram: X ray of blood vessels taken after injection of dye.

Ascites: Abnormal fluid in the abdomen.

Benign tumor: Abnormal growth that is not a cancer. It cannot spread to other parts of the body. It can sometimes cause problems because of its location.

Biochemical markers: Proteins that are detected in abnormal amounts in the blood or at the site of a cancer. They are used to diagnose and follow some cancers. Even with today's technology, only some cancers have biochemical markers that are useful in the care of patients.

Biological therapy: Treatment by stimulation of the body's immune defense system; immunotherapy

Biopsy: Removal and examination under the microscope of a piece of tissue from a living person.

Bone marrow: Soft substance in the center of bones; the place where blood is made.

Cancer: A general term for over two hundred diseases characterized by abnormal and uncontrolled growth of cells. The mass, or tumor, can invade and destroy surrounding normal tissues. The cancer cells can spread through the blood or lymph system to start new cancers in other parts of the body.

Carcinoma: Cancer that begins in tissue that lines an organ or duct.

CAT scan: A sophisticated X-ray that shows cross-sectional views of the area pictured (see Appendix E).

Cell: The unit structure of all living tissue.

Chemotherapy: Treatment with anti-cancer drugs.

CSF (Colony Stimulating Factor): A substance produced by the healthy body to regulate the number and function of blood cells. They can also be produced artificially, and studies are underway to see if they will help cancer patients tolerate cancer therapy and fight cancer. If effective, CSF may help overcome some of the most serious complications of cancer therapy, including susceptibility to bacterial infection and risk of bleeding. CSF may enable patients to receive higher, more effective amounts of therapy.

Cure: When doctors talk of a cancer cure, they usually mean that there is no detectable sign of cancer and the person has the same life expectancy as if he or she never had cancer. Sometimes doctors use the word "cure" when there is no evidence of cancer for at least five years. This is because for most cancers five years is a fairly reliable time after which the chance of recurrence is extremely low. Some cancers can be called "cured" in one year, other cancers cannot be called cured even after five years with no sign of cancer. Every cancer is different. You will need to find out what your doctors mean when they talk about "curing" your type of cancer.

Cyst: Sac containing fluid and/or solid material; usually benign, but can be malignant.

Debulking: Procedure to remove as much of the cancer as possible; reducing the "bulk" of the cancer.

Diagnosis: The name of your illness.

Estrogen: Female sex hormone.

Fine-needle aspiration: Using a needle to biopsy a tumor through the skin.

Hepatic: Related to the liver.

Hormone status: The hormone status of an individual's cancer is determined by sophisticated tests done on a piece of the cancer. The tests indicate which hormones may affect the cancer cell. Hormone status can only be determined for a few types of cancer.

Hormonal therapy: The use of hormones to treat cancer.

Immune system: White blood cells and antibodies that protect the body by attacking foreign substances.

Immunotherapy: Treatment by stimulation of the body's immune defense system.

Induction therapy: The initial treatment to eliminate or control cancer.

Interferons: Proteins produced by the body to help fight infection; they have been found to have some anti-cancer properties.

Interleukins: Substances that are produced by the healthy body to help in the controlled production of blood cells as well as the body's immune responses. These sugar-protein molecules can be made artificially, and studies are underway to determine if giving these substances to cancer patients will help the patient's own body fight the cancer.

Kaposi's sarcoma: Before the AIDS epidemic, Kaposi's sarcoma (classic Kaposi's sarcoma) was known as a slow-growing cancer of the skin of the legs. Kaposi's sarcoma in the person with AIDS involves widespread cancer of the skin, and frequently spreads to the lymph nodes, gastrointestinal tract, and lungs. AIDS patients with Kaposi's sarcoma seem to do better overall than those AIDS patients without Kaposi's sarcoma.

Leukemia: Cancer of the white blood cells.

Living will: A written document that outlines how much you would want doctors to do to prolong your life (with medicines and machines) if you were critically ill with little hope of recovery.

Localized: Limited to the site of origin, no evidence of spread.

Lymph fluid: Clear fluid formed throughout the body, which flows in the lymph system, is filtered in the lymph nodes, and then is added to the blood.

Lymph nodes: Rounded bean-shaped organs that make some of the white blood cells (lymphocytes and monocytes) and filter the lymph fluid before it enters the blood; they vary in size from a pinhead to the size of an olive. We have thousands of them throughout our body, the most obvious ones in the neck (cervical region), armpit (axillary region), and groin (inguinal region); they may become a place to which cancer spreads.

Lymphatic system: A circulation system, like the blood system, that carries lymph throughout the body. Lymph is a colorless fluid that carries infection-fighting cells. The lymph organs include the lymph nodes, spleen, and thymus.

Lymphoma: Cancer of the lymph system.

Malignant: Cancerous.

Mastectomy: Surgical removal of the breast.

Metastasis (plural = metastases): Cancer cells that have spread from their original site.

Metastasize: To spread.

Monoclonal antibody therapy: A new technique being investigated for treating cancer, involving very specific antibodies that will react specifically with the cancer cells.

Multiple myeloma: Cancer of the plasma cells in the bone marrow

Neoplasm: Tumor, abnormal growth of tissue; may be benign or malignant.

Nodule: Lump, tumor; may be benign or malignant.

Non-Hodgkin's lymphoma: A type of cancer of the lymph system. Intermediate and high-grade non-Hodgkin's lymphoma are the faster-growing forms of this type of cancer. This type of cancer occurs in people without AIDS (Acquired Immune Deficiency Syndrome). However, people with AIDS have an increased risk of developing intermediate and high-grade non-Hodgkin's lymphoma. In the patients with AIDS, their lymphoma tends to have a poor response to treatment and tends to recur after treatment.

Oncologist: Doctor specializing in cancer diagnosis and treatment.

Oncology: The branch of medicine dealing with cancer.

Ostomy: Surgical opening in the skin, allowing connection to an internal organ for drainage.

Pathologist: Doctor specialized in diagnosing disease by looking at tissue directly, under the microscope and with other technology.

Palliative: Treatment for comfort, not cure.

Platelet: Type of blood cell in the circulation, very important in clotting (mechanism to stop bleeding).

Primary lesion: Place where the cancer first started.

Prognosis: Prediction of how well you will do.

Protocol: Description of the treatment steps (the "recipe").

Radiation therapy: Treatment using radioactive substances.

Radiotherapist: Physician who specializes in the treatment of disease by means of radiation therapy.

Receptors: Receptors are proteins on the surface of all cells that bind with available complementary proteins. Some receptors are found only on normal cells, some are found on both normal and cancer cells, and some are found only on cancer cells. Sophisticated tests can now identify and quantitate the presence of some receptors.

Receptor expression: Receptor expression refers to how many specific receptors are found on the surface of a cancer cell, and how effective they are at doing their job. Determinations of receptor expression may help determine the most effective therapy, and will hopefully lead to the development of cancer therapy that only kills cancer cells and leaves normal cells alone.

Recurrence: Reappearance of the same cancer after a period when there was no evidence of cancer.

Remission: Partial or complete shrinkage of cancer.

Residual disease (or cancer, or tumor): Remaining cancer.

Sarcoma: Cancer of the soft tissue (muscles, nerves, tendons, blood vessels, or bones.

Spleen: An organ in the left upper abdomen that is part of the lymph system. It helps to remove old red blood cells, produce white blood cells, and store blood.

Staging: Evaluation to see how far the cancer has spread.

Tissue: Group of similar cells.

Tumor Necrosis Factor: Proteins that are released by certain white blood cells in response to bacterial infection. Laboratory tests have shown these proteins to be lethal to some cancer cells. Studies are underway to evaluate the safety and efficacy of TNF's in cancer patients.

Tumors: Abnormal masses of tissue that may be either benign or malignant (cancerous).

Uterus: Womb; organ in which unborn child grows.

APPENDIX B

Annotated Bibliography

UNDERSTANDING CANCER. GETTING INTO THE MEDICAL SYSTEM (CHAPTERS 1 AND 2)

There are numerous books that discuss the medical aspects of cancer in greater detail. Few of them can be read cover-to-cover, but they serve as excellent references for more in-depth explanations of specific questions or areas of oncology. As oncology is a rapidly changing field, it is very important to check copyright dates. Statistics about cancers and specifics about treatment may be woefully misleading if the book is a few years old. *Everyone's Guide to Cancer Therapy: How Cancer Is Diagnosed, Treated, and Managed Day to Day* by Malin Dollinger, M.D., et al. (Kansas City, Mo., and New York, Andrews and McMeel, 1991, 624 pages) is an excellent, comprehensive resource written for the layperson. It reviews in clear detail the basics of cancer diagnosis and treatment; working with the healthcare team (doctors, nurses, support groups); the physical and emotional aspects of cancer diagnosis, treatment, and survival; and the common cancers. *Choices: Realistic Alternatives in Cancer Treatment* by Marion Morra and Eva Potts (New York, Avon Books, 1987, 954 pages) is another excellent comprehensive resource for the layperson, written in question-answer format.

Two well-respected textbooks are *Cancer: Principles and Practice of Oncology,* edited by Vincent T. DeVita, Jr., et al. (3d ed.) (Philadelphia, Lippincott, 1990) and *Comprehensive Textbook of Oncology,* by A. R. Moosa et al. (2d ed.). (Baltimore, Williams and Wilkins, 1991). These two books are medical texts written for the physician. They are mammoth volumes, written in technical language, assuming a sophisticated medical background. There are also a number of oncology journals that are available for review in medical school libraries. These tend to be quite technical and sophisticated.

PRACTICAL ISSUES (CHAPTER 3)

There are many issues common to all cancer patients, and other issues that are specific to patients in certain situations or receiving certain treatments. Dollinger's *Everyone's Guide to Cancer Therapy* is a very useful resource for understanding and dealing with treatment side effects, pain, nutrition, and exercise. Marion Morra and Eve Potts's *Choices* is also a useful resource, replete with explanations and suggestions. *Charting the Journey: An Almanac of Practical Resources for Cancer Survivors,* edited by Mullan, M.D., Hoffman, J.D., and the Editors of Consumer Reports Books (New York, Consumers Union, 1990) was devised by the National Coalition for Cancer Survivorship. It is written in clear language for the layperson, focusing on the practical aspects of surviving after the initial diagnosis and treatment and later after treatment is complete. It includes a discussion of legal, financial, and insurance problems. *Surviving Cancer: A Practical Guide for Those Fighting to Win* by Danette G. Kauffman (Washington, D.C., Acropolis, 1989) is a nice guide to dealing with practical and emotional issues of cancer. A unique strength of this book is a thorough listing of resources at the end of each section. *I Can Cope: Staying Healthy With Cancer* by Judi Johnson and Linda Klein (Minneapolis, Minn., DCI Publishing, 1988) is an outgrowth of the American Cancer Society's "I Can Cope" program. Through the stories of a handful of cancer patients who are coping with their illnesses, the book relates the philosophies and tools advanced by the "I Can Cope" support groups. *Beauty and Cancer: A Woman's Guide to Looking Great while Experiencing Side Effects of Cancer Therapy* by Noyes and Mel-lody (Los Angeles, Calif., AC Press, 1988) is an upbeat resource for women, devoted to the cosmetic changes of therapy. It presents many ways to cope with the physical changes that can occur, encour-aging you to feel attractive and "whole" despite the physical and emotional changes of cancer therapy. It supplies medically sound advice on skin care, makeup, nutrition, exercise, and nail care. This book introduces you to fashionable hair and clothes alternatives to fit your special needs. *Winning the Chemo Battle* by Joyce Slayton Mitch-ell (New York, Norton, 1991) is a very readable account of a writer's experience with chemotherapy. She juxtaposes her own story with basic information and advice about the experience of receiving che-motherapy. *Vital Signs: A Young Doctor's Struggle with Cancer* written by the co-founder of the National Coalition of Cancer Survivorship, is the moving story of a doctor coming to terms with what it means to be a patient. *When Someone You Love Has Cancer* by Dana Rae Pome-roy (Santa Monica, Calif., IBS Press, 1991) is a reassuring and practi-cal guide for the family and friends of a cancer patient.

THE EMOTIONAL ADJUSTMENT (CHAPTERS 4 AND 5)

The Road Back to Health: Coping with the Emotional Aspects of Cancer by Neil A. Fiore, Ph.D. (Berkeley, Calif., Celestial Arts, 1990) is a book for cancer patients and their families, written by a psychothera-pist who was treated for cancer in 1974. He reviews and assists with the emotional adjustment to all stages of the cancer experience. He discusses the doctor-patient relationship, how to be an active patient, how to cope with treatments, and how to deal with your own emo-tions, as well as how to communicate effectively with family and medical staff. *Fighting Cancer* by Annette and Richard Bloch (Kansas City, MO, RA Bloch Cancer Foundation, 1985) is a forceful, straight-forward book whose purpose is to encourage you to get the best care you can, as well as adopt a hopeful attitude even in the face of unfa-vorable statistics. It is available free of charge by writing to The Cancer Hot Line, Annette and Richard Bloch, 4410 Main Street, Kan-sas City, MO 64111. *Why Me? Coping with Grief, Loss, and Change,* by Rabbi Pesach Krauss (New York 1988) is a readable and moving book that teaches you to grow in the face of crisis, and to have hope in the face of pain and despair. Rabbi Krauss has lived with pain and loss himself, and has worked with cancer patients at Memorial Sloan-Kettering Cancer Center. In *And a Time to Live: Toward Emotional Well-Being during the Crisis of Cancer,* (New York, 1978) R. C. Cantor analyzes problems that arise with emotions and relationships and offers advice on how best to deal with these changes. *You Can't Afford the Luxury of a Negative Thought* by John-Roger & McWilliams (Los Angeles, Calif., 1990) is a large volume of inspirational thoughts and sayings. *Making Miracles: An Exploration into the Dynamics of Self-healing* by P.C. Roud (New York, Warner, 1990) is another very readable book that encourages hope when a person is faced with life-threatening illness. Eleven people with "terminal illness" who outlived all expectations discuss their approach to their illnesses and their lives. *The Road Less Traveled* by M. Scott Peck (New York, Simon & Schuster, 1978) is a popular book by a psychiatrist that offers a path to self-awareness and spiritual growth.

APPENDIX C

▬

Resources for the Newly Diagnosed Patient

NCI (NATIONAL CANCER INSTITUTE)

The National Cancer Institute provides a Cancer Information Service (CIS). 1-800-4-CANCER is a toll-free number answered by paid professional information specialists. They are prepared to answer questions about cancer or direct you to the place or person where you can get your answer. They have a large number of informational booklets available free of charge. After you are first diagnosed with cancer, you may want to request the booklet pertaining to your type of cancer entitled "What You Need to Know about Cancer." Two other booklets that are helpful in the beginning are "Taking Time" and "Facing Forward." You can request a list of all of NCI's publications. They can also provide you with the most recent printing of PDQ (Physician Data Query). This is a frequently updated summary of the work being done on your type of cancer. There is an edition for patients and an edition for physicians (you are welcome to both editions).

THE AMERICAN CANCER SOCIETY (ACS)

The American Cancer Society has national and local offices. You can obtain the telephone number of the local office from your oncologist or the Yellow Pages. They have trained volunteers, many of whom have dealt with cancer themselves, to answer questions. They can usually provide information and referrals (lists of local oncologists, support groups, supply stores).

THE NATIONAL COALITION FOR CANCER SURVIVOR-SHIP (NCCS)

The National Coalition for Cancer Survivorship is a growing movement, focusing on issues of importance to cancer survivors. They have a quarterly newsletter, *The Networker,* available by writing:

> National Coalition for Cancer Survivorship
> 1010 Wayne Avenue
> 5th Floor
> Silver Springs, M.D. 20910
> (301) 585-2616

SOCIAL SERVICES

The social service department of your local hospital is usually well-versed in all the services available in your community (support groups, local supply stores, local support services, local treatment facilities).

THE OFFICE OF YOUR ONCOLOGIST

The staff of your oncologist is familiar with most of the needs and problems that you will have, as well as services available in the local community.

━━━

Sample Medication List

Week of _____

Time	MEDICINE	Dose	Sun	Mon	Tue	Wed	Thu	Fri	Sat

APPENDIX E

Explanation of Common Tests

The evaluation and treatment of cancer involves tests. Tests are used to:

- Determine the extent of your cancer at the time of your original diagnosis
- Uncover any coexisting or related problems at the time of your original diagnosis
- Establish a baseline for your followup studies
- Monitor the response of your cancer to the therapy
- Identify and evaluate any complications that may develop during treatment
- Evaluate for recurrent disease if treatment has rendered you free of cancer

The risk of complications for each test may vary from patient to patient depending on:

- Which technique is used by the lab
- The experience of the people administering and interpreting the test
- Your medical condition

Your doctors are balancing the risk, inconvenience, and expense of each test against the benefit of the information gained. You are taking a risk if you decline or modify a test, since the test may provide information that is valuable to your health. Invasive tests are riskier than non-invasive tests. Tests that require more X ray exposure carry more long-term risk than tests that require less X ray exposure. Contrast (dye that is ingested, injected, or given by enema) can cause problems in susceptible people.

An estimate of the time it takes to undergo a test does not include the time you wait in the reception area, nor the time it takes to set up the test. The time required for the test will vary depending upon:

- The speed of the specific equipment used
- Your medical condition (how easy it is to find a vein for injection, how well you can hold still or hold a deep breath)
- How good the pictures or samples are (if the pictures are fuzzy, they will have to be retaken; if the biopsy specimen is too small, it will have to be redone)

When you schedule a test, be sure that you are clear about:

- The time that you are supposed to arrive for your test
- The place that you are supposed to go for your test
- Any dietary restrictions prior to the test
- Whether or not you will need someone to accompany you to or from the test
- Any special medication that is supposed to be taken or preparation that is supposed to be completed prior to the test
- Whether you are supposed to take all of your regular medicines on the day of your test

Make sure the people doing the test are aware if you have

- A history of asthma or allergies, especially allergies to iodine or latex

- A tendency towards claustrophobia
- Any chance of being pregnant

The results of your test are sent to the doctor who ordered the test (usually your oncologist), who will then review the results with you. Expect a delay between the completion of a test and the availability of a final report. Preliminary reports are sometimes provided. You can ask the people doing the test how long it usually takes to get the final results of your tests. Do not assume that "no news is good news." If you have not heard the results of your test, have the doctor's office review the results with you.

Angiogram = arteriogram = contrast vascular study

An angiogram shows the distribution and condition of blood vessels in the area tested. Using gentle sedation and local anesthetic, a catheter (thin plastic tube) is inserted into an artery. Usually the large artery in the groin is used as the entry site, although occasionally another artery is used. Dye is injected into an artery supplying the area to be studied, and rapid-sequence X rays are then taken. There is minimal discomfort other than having to lie still on a hard table. Angiography is a higher-risk study but is still relatively safe in skilled hands. (Average time: ninety minutes)

    cerebral angiogram = vessels to the brain
    coronary angiogram = vessels to the heart
    pulmonary angiogram = vessels to the lung
    renal angiogram = vessels to the kidney
    visceral angiogram = vessels to the organs in the abdomen

Barium enema = BE

This is an X ray of the colon and rectum. Barium is given by enema into the rectum, where it outlines the inner surface of the colon and rectum. If it is an "air contrast barium enema," air is introduced after the barium. You may feel distended and uncomfortable as you hold the barium and air in your colon while the X rays are taken. (Average time: twenty minutes)

BONE MARROW BIOPSY

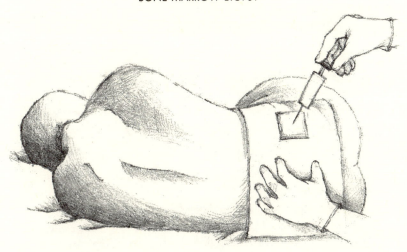

Barium swallow

This is an X ray of the pharynx (throat) and esophagus. A barium-containing liquid, and sometimes a barium-containing wafer, is swallowed. X rays are taken while you are swallowing, to show the contractions of the esophagus as well as to outline the inner surface of the pharynx and esophagus. Pictures may be taken while you are in different positions. Some people find the taste of the barium solution unpleasant. (Average time: five minutes)

Bone marrow biopsy

This is a test to obtain a sample of bone marrow for analysis. The sample is usually obtained from the marrow in your hip or your sternum (breast bone). While you are lying on an exam table or hospital bed, the skin and bone are made numb using local anesthetic. A special needle is then put into the bone and a sample of the marrow is withdrawn. There is the sensation of painless pressure as the needle is pushed through the bone into the marrow. There is pain for a second or two as the marrow is removed. You may be sore, as if you had a bruise, at the site of the biopsy for a few days. The entire procedure takes ten minutes.

Bone scan

A bone scan is a picture of all of the bones in the body, using a small amount of injected radioactive substance. Abnormalities show up as an area of increased or decreased radioactivity. You receive an injection in your vein containing the radioactive substance one and one-half to two and one-half hours prior to the scan. Some people find it uncomfortable to lie still on the hard scanner table for the thirty minutes it takes to do the scan.

CT scan = CAT scan = computerized axial tomography = computed tomography

This is a sophisticated X ray that shows cross-sectional views of the area pictured. In many cases, CT scans are used instead of surgery to help stage and follow cancer (see Chapter 1). Sometimes contrast has to be taken by mouth prior to the study. Injection of dye into a vein during the test is usually required. You may be asked to hold your breath for a few moments while some of the X rays are taken. You will be alone in the room during the X rays, but you will be able to talk with the technicians throughout the test via a two-way intercom. People with a tendency towards claustrophobia may feel anxious during this test. Medication can be given to help this anxiety, so discuss this with your doctor. Some people find it uncomfortable to lie still in one position for the duration of the test. Some areas may be scanned without contrast, and then scanned again after contrast is given. Sometimes your situation requires repeating the scan with thinner slices. It takes approximately thirty minutes to do *one* scan of the head, or the chest, or the abdomen, or a limb.

Cystogram

This is an X ray of your urinary bladder. Dye is introduced into your bladder through a urinary catheter. It is uncomfortable for a few seconds as the catheter is placed in your bladder. Some people find it uncomfortable to hold a full bladder as the pictures are taken. (Average time: fifteen minutes)

Gallium scan

This is a picture of the body using a small amount of radioactive substance. Any areas of inflammation or dividing cells show up on the scan as an area of increased radioactivity. First, you receive an injection containing the radioactive tracer in a vein on your arm. Twenty-four hours after the injection, and again forty-eight hours after the injection, you lie still on a hard table as the scanner makes the pictures. It takes thirty minutes to do each scan.

IVP = intravenous pyelogram

This is an X ray of the kidneys. A dye is given in your vein, after which X rays are taken of your kidneys as the dye is excreted. If your kidney function is normal, the test takes approximately twenty minutes. If there are certain kidney problems, X rays may need to be taken periodically for a few hours. You may be requested to return for more X rays later in the day or the next day. People who may have multiple myeloma, allergy to the contrast, or kidney failure should be sure that the radiologists are aware of these conditions.

Liver-spleen scan

This is a picture of your liver and spleen, using a small amount of radioactive substance. First, you receive an injection containing the radioactive tracer in a vein in your arm. Twenty minutes later, you lie still on a hard table for twenty minutes as the scanner makes the picture.

Lumbar puncture = spinal tap

This is a simple procedure to obtain spinal fluid for analysis. After an area in your back is made numb with local anesthetic, a needle is inserted to get a sample of spinal fluid. If you have a lot of curvature or arthritis, this procedure is sometimes done under an X ray machine. You have to hold still during the test. It takes five to ten minutes, and there is usually minimal if any discomfort during the procedure. A few people will complain of a headache afterwards. Discuss the risks with your doctor.

LUMBAR PUNCTURE

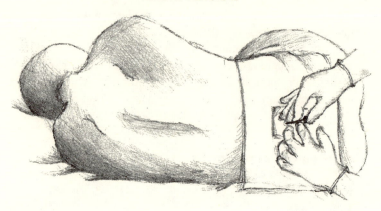

With the patient lying comfortably curled up, the area is cleaned, then draped with sterile paper. The entry site is first anesthetized with local anesthetic. The spinal needle is then introduced and spinal fluid obtained.

Lymphogram = lymphangiogram

This is an X ray of the lymph nodes in your pelvis and abdomen. Dye is injected into the veins in your feet, after which X rays are taken of your pelvis and abdomen. The first X rays only take a few minutes, but you may be asked to return for X rays twenty-four and forty-eight hours after the injection of dye. It is uncomfortable when the dye is injected. The test involves a risk of inflammation of the lymph channels.

Mammogram

A mammogram is a picture of the breast using low-dose X rays. It is used to screen for breast cancers too small to be felt. Mammography is also used after a lump is discovered to help determine if the lump is suspicious for cancer. A mammogram is not foolproof; if a lump is suspicious, it should be biopsied even if the mammogram is normal. To have a mammogram, you stand in front of a small table on which your breast is placed. A special plate then flattens the breast against the table, and the X ray is taken. Large-breasted women sometimes find the breast compression uncomfortable. Small-breasted women sometimes find leaning their rib cage against the table uncomfortable. However, the test takes only a few minutes.

MRI scan = NMR scan = magnetic resonance imaging scan

This is an imaging technique that uses a magnetic field and radio waves instead of X rays. The pictures obtained are quite detailed. People with a tendency towards claustrophobia may feel anxious during this test. Medication can be given to minimize this anxiety, so discuss this with your doctor. MRI scans take longer to do than CT scans. Some people find it uncomfortable to lie still in one position for the duration of the test. During the test, there is a loud tapping sound. You may request earplugs to minimize the discomfort from this noise. (Average time: thirty minutes for a scan of the head, sixty minutes for other scans)

Myelogram

This is an X ray test to show the spinal cord. Dye is injected into the spinal fluid (see *lumbar puncture* in this Appendix), after which you lie prone on a table that is tilted in various angles to allow the dye to flow around to all parts of the spinal cord. X rays are taken in different positions. There may be discomfort associated with the spinal tap. A few people develop a headache after the procedure. (Average time: forty-five minutes for one section of the spine, longer if the entire spine is to be evaluated. You will have to remain lying down or semi-erect for a while after the test is completed. Frequently, a CT scan is done after the myelogram.)

Plain radiography = plain X ray = plain film = X ray

This is a standard X ray. It involves low-dose radiation exposure and takes a few minutes. It is generally painless, although some positioning requirements may cause discomfort. (Average time: one to five minutes)

Ultrasound

This is a non-invasive, fast, and safe technique which uses sound waves to create pictures of the inside of your body. First, gel is placed on the skin overlying the area to be evaluated. Then a

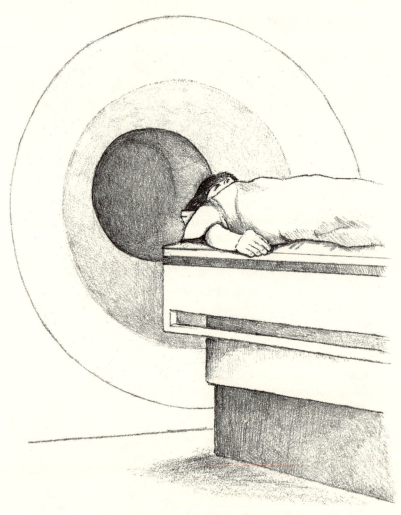

MAGNETIC RESONANCE IMAGING SCAN

transducer, which looks like a wand or a microphone, is placed on the gel and slowly slid along your skin. Pelvic ultrasounds require a full bladder, which can be uncomfortable, during the test. You will have to lie still for the short time required for the test, or hold your breath for a few seconds during the test. (Average time: thirty minutes for the abdomen, fifteen minutes for the breast)

UGI = upper GI = upper gastrointestinal series

This is an X ray of the stomach. A contrast-containing solution is swallowed, during and after which X rays are taken. If additional pictures are taken after the contrast passes from the stomach into the small bowel (intestines), the additional X rays are called a "small bowel follow-through" (SBFT). You will lie on a special table that tilts. Some people find the taste of the solution that you drink to be unpleasant. (Average time: sixty minutes for an UGI, up to five hours for a SBFT)

APPENDIX F

Medical Abbreviations

You will come across medical abbreviations on your prescriptions, instructions, or insurance forms. Here is a list of frequently used abbreviations. They are often abbreviated Latin words so whenever you are not sure about an abbreviation, check it with your doctor's office.

a.c. = before meals
ad lib = as desired, as much as you want
b.i.d. = b.d. = two times a day (check if they want you to take the medicine or treatment every twelve hours, or just any two times during the day)
aa = a = of each
c. = with
ext. = extract
fl = fluid
gtt = a drop
gtts = drops
hgb = hemoglobin (related to red blood cell count)

h.s. = at bedtime
I.M. = intramuscular = in the muscle
I.V. = intravenous = in the vein
kg = kilogram
N.P.O. = nothing by mouth = fasting
p.c. = after meals
p.o. = per os = given by mouth
p.r.n. = as needed (for example, "every six hours p.r.n." means
        that you can take the medicine as often as every six hours,
        but you would only take the medicine if you needed it)
Q. = every (for example, "Q. 8 hrs" means every 8 hours)
q.a.m. = every morning
q.d. = every day
Q.h. = every hour
q.h.s. = every evening
q.i.d. = four times a day
q.o.d. = every other day
s = without
sig = write = let it be labeled
sub q = under the skin
suppos. = suppository
t.i.d. = three times a day

APPENDIX G

Sample Living Will

TO MY FAMILY, MY PHYSICIAN, MY LAWYER AND ALL OTHERS WHOM IT MAY CONCERN

Death is as much a reality as birth, growth, and aging—it is the one certainty of life. In anticipation of decisions that may have to be made about my own dying and as an expression of my right to refuse treatment, I, _____
(print name)
being of sound mind, make this statement of my wishes and instructions concerning treatment.

By means of this document, which I intend to be legally binding, I direct my physician and other care providers, my family, and any surrogate designated by me or appointed by a court, to carry out my wishes. If I become unable, by reason of physical or mental incapacity, to make decisions about my medical care, let this document provide the guidance and authority needed to make any and all such decisions.

If I am permanently unconscious or there is no reasonable expectation of my recovery from a seriously incapacitating or lethal illness or condition, I do not wish to be kept alive by artificial means. I request that I be given all care necessary to keep me comfortable and free of pain, even if pain-relieving medications may hasten my death, and I direct that no life-sustaining treatment be provided except as I or my surrogate specifically authorize.

This request may appear to place a heavy responsibility upon you, but by making this decision according to my strong convictions, I intend to ease that burden. I am acting after careful consideration and with understanding of the consequences of your carrying out my wishes. *List optional specific provisions in the space below.*

Durable Power of Attorney for Health Care Decisions

(Cross out if you do not wish to use this section)

To effect my wishes, I designate, _____
residing at, _____
(phone #), _____
(or if he or she shall for any reason fail to act, _____
residing at, _____
(phone #) _____
as my health care surrogate—that is, my attorney-in-fact regarding any and all health care decisions to be made for me, including the decision to refuse life-sustaining treatment—if I am unable to make such decisions myself. This power shall remain effective during and not be affected by my subsequent illness, disability or incapacity. My surrogate shall have authority to interpret my Living Will, and shall make decisions about my health care as specified in my instructions or, when my wishes are not clear, as the surrogate believes to be in my best interests. I release and agree to hold harmless my health care surrogate from any and all claims whatsoever arising from decisions made in good faith in the exercise of this power.

I sign this document know-
ingly, voluntarily, and after careful deliberation, this _____ day of
_____ , 19 _____ .

_____
(signature)

Address _____

_____

I do hereby certify that the within
document was executed and ac-
knowledged before me by the
principal   this _____ day   of
_____ , 19 _____ .

_____
Notary Public

Witness _____
Printed Name _____
Address _____

_____

Witness _____
Printed Name _____
Address _____

_____

Copies of this document have
been given to:

This Living Will expresses my personal treatment preferences.
The fact that I may have also executed a declaration in the form
recommended by state law should not be construed to limit or con-
tradict this Living Will, which is an expression of my common-law
and constitutional rights.

(Optional) my Living Will
is registered with Concern for Dying (Registry No. _____)

Distributed by Concern for Dying,
250 West 57th Street, New York, NY 10107 (212) 246-6962

Index

relaxation, as supplemental therapy, 30
religion, 79, 98
remission:
    definition of, 19
    partial (response), 19, 40
    spontaneous, 4
    treatment options and, 40
risk factors, 6–8, 9
    chemotherapy and, 69
    cure and, 40
    diet as, 8
    family and, 7, 89
    individuality of, 32
    tests and, 116–17
    treatment options and, 31–33, 40
    work as, 69
    see also causes

sarcoma, 9, 10
SBFT (small bowel follow-through), 125
scans:
    bone, 120
    CAT (CT), 17, 120, 123
    gallium, 121
    liver-spleen, 121
    MRI (NMR), 123, 124
    surgical evaluation vs., 14–15
school, see work and school
second opinions, 44
self-blame, 6–7, 80, 88, 91
self-cure, 91–92
self-help, 92, 93, 98
sex, 89–90
side effects:
    decrease in, 33–34
    hypnosis and, 93
    of radiation, 22
    response to therapy and, 34
    treatment options and, 31–32, 40
    weight changes as, 64–65, 66–67
social services, 114
Society for the Right to Die, 75
sperm, banking of, 36
spinal tap (lumbar puncture), 121–22, 123
spreading of cancer, see metastasis
staging, 13–18
    definition of, 13
    methods of, 13–14
    options in, 14–15
    prognosis and, 14, 15
    purposes of, 14
    tests in, 13–17
    timing of, 18
    treatment options and, 15, 18, 21
standard therapy, 24, 27
stress:
    causes of cancer and, 7–8
    management of, 63, 91–92
supplemental therapy, 30

supply stores, 114
support groups, 18, 30, 90, 98
    definition of, 86
    denial and, 79
    locations of, 87, 114
    participation in, 86–87
surgery:
    radiation and, 22
    staging and, 14
    as treatment option, 20
survival, xx
symptoms, 99–100

team concept in doctoring, 47
test results:
    communication with doctor about, 118
    lack of control over, 96
    negative, 16, 17
    positive, 16–17
tests, 116–25
    allergies and, 118
    blood, 9, 48–49
    claustrophobia and, 118, 123
    communication with doctor about, 51, 100,
        117
    complications from, 116–17
    dental exam, 54–55
    dietary restrictions for, 117
    fertility and, 35–36
    leaves of absence for, 68
    marker, 18
    medicines and, 117
    for metastasis, 15–16
    non-cancer-related, 50–51
    physical exam, 14, 50
    pregnancy and, 118
    purposes of, 116
    rechecking of, after treatment, 15
    risk factors in, 116–17
    in staging, 13–17
    timing of, 50–51, 117
therapy, see treatment
timing:
    of staging, 18
    of tests, 50–51, 117
    of treatment, 34–35
treatment, 19–42
    cure and, 4, 19, 27, 32
    diet and, 65
    early, 18
    fears about, 42
    improvements in, xxi, 5
    leaves of absence for, 68–69
    length of, 30
    location of, 30
    mental reactions to, 97
    purposes of, 19
    regulation of, 28
    supplemental, 30

DATE DUE

12/8/97			
12/8/97			
GAYLORD			PRINTED IN U.S.A.